AIR FRYER COOKBOOK

Series 7

This Book Includes : "The Complete Air Fryer Cookbook + The Air Fryer Recipes"

By Denise White

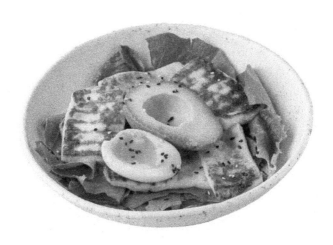

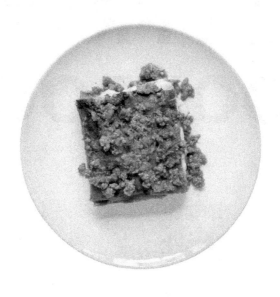

THE COMPLETE AIR FRYER COOKBOOK

Table of Contents

Introduction.. 16

Recipes 17

  1.Basil Tomato Frittata.. 17

  2.Italian Breakfast Frittata 18

  3.Healthy Baked Omelets 19

  4.Easy Egg Casserole 21

  5.Flavor Packed Breakfast Casserole 22

  6.Vegetable Sausage Egg Bake 23

  7.Ham Egg Brunch Bake 24

  8.Cheese Broccoli Bake 25

  9.Sweet Potato Frittata 26

  10.Toasty Grilled Chicken with Cauliflower and Garlic Butter ... 28

  11.Garlic Turkey 29

  12.Sweet and Sticky Turkey Wings 30

  13.Tofu and Cabbage Plate 31

  14.Thai Fish 31

  15.Chicken with Parsnips 32

  16.Salmon Salad with Boiled Eggs 33

  17.Tomato Mint Soup 34

  18.Fried Cauliflower Rice.. 35

  19.Baked Salmon 36

  20.Prosciutto-Wrapped Parmesan Asparagus............. 36

  21.Bacon-Wrapped Jalapeño Poppers 37

  22.Garlic Parmesan Chicken Wings............................ 38

23.Spicy Buffalo Chicken Dip 38

24.Bacon Jalapeño Cheese Bread............................... 39

25.Pizza Rolls 40

27.Bacon Cheeseburger Dip...................................... 41

28.Pork Rind Tortillas.. 42

29.Mozzarella Sticks 43

30.Bacon-Wrapped Onion Rings 43

31.Crusted Chicken Tenders 44

32.Air Fryer Chicken Parmesan................................. 45

33.Chicken Bbq Recipe from Peru 45

34.Ricotta and Parsley Stuffed Turkey Breasts 46

35.Cheesy Turkey-Rice with Broccoli 48

36.Jerk Chicken Wings 48

37. Brazilian Mini Turkey Pies.................................. 50

38.Pork Taquitos... 51

39.Panko-breaded pork chops 51

40.Apricot glazed pork tenderloins 52

41.Barbecue Flavored Pork Ribs 53

42.Balsamic Glazed Pork Chops 54

43.Rustic Pork Ribs... 54

44.Keto Parmesan Crusted Pork Chops 55

45.Crispy Fried Pork Chops the Southern Way.......... 56

46.Scrumptious Rib-Eye Steak.................................. 57

47.Air Fryer Toast Oven Sticky Pork Ribs 57

48.Coriander Lamb with Pesto' N Mint Dip 58

49.Cumin-Sichuan Lamb Bbq with Dip 60

50.Garlic Lemon-Wine on Lamb Steak...................... 61

51.Garlic-Rosemary Lamb Bbq.................................. 61

52.Maras Pepper Lamb Kebab Recipe from Turkey ... 62

53.Saffron Spiced Rack of Lamb 63

54.Shepherd's Pie Made Of Ground Lamb................. 63

55.Simple Lamb Bbq with Herbed Salt 65

56.Greek Lamb Meatballs 65

57.Lamb Gyro 66

58.Masala Galette 68

59.Potato Samosa 68

60.Vegetable Kebab 70

61.Sago Galette 71

62.Stuffed Capsicum Baskets 71

63.Baked Macaroni Pasta 73

64.Macaroni Samosa 74

65.Burritos 75

66.Cheese and Bean Enchiladas................................ 78

67.Veg Memo's 79

68.Yummy Pollock 81

69.Honey Sea Bass.. 82

70.Tilapia Sauce and Chives 83

71.Tilapia Coconut 83

72.Catfish fillets special 84

73.Tasty French Cod... 85

74.Scampi Shrimp and Chips 86

75.Gambas 'Pil' with Sweet Potato 87

76.Fried Hot Prawns with Cocktail Sauce 88

77.Crispy Air-fryer Coconut Prawns......................... 89

78.Crispy Crabstick Crackers 91

79.Wasabi Crab Cakes... 91

80.Flourless Truly Crispy Calamari Rings 93

81.Scallops Wrapped in Bacon................................. 94

82.Tilapia Fillet with Vegetables.............................. 94

83.Shrimps in the Pumpkin 94

84.Shrimp Strogonoff.. 95

85.Pumpkin Shrimp with Catupiry 96

86.Fricassee of Jamila Shrimps.. 97

87.Fried Beach Shrimps... 98

88.Fried Shrimp without Flour 99

89.Shrimps with Garlic and Oil 99

90.Breaded Prawns... 100

Conclusion 111

THE AIR FRYER RECIPES

Table of Contents

Introduction...116

Recipes..117

  1.Mini Veggie Quiche Cups...117

  2.Lemon Blueberry Muffins...119

  3.Baked Breakfast Donuts...121

  4.Blueberry Almond Muffins.......................................122

  5.Feta Broccoli Frittata...123

  6.Creamy Spinach Quiche..125

  7.Turkey and Quinoa Stuffed Peppers.......................125

  8.Curried Chicken, Chickpeas and Raito Salad.........127

  9.Balsamic Vinaigrette on Roasted Chicken.............129

  10.Chicken Pasta Parmesan......................................130

  11.Chicken and White Bean.......................................131

  12.Chicken Thighs with Butternut Squash.................133

  13.Cajun Rice & Chicken..134

  14.Vegetable Lover's Chicken Soup..........................136

  15.Coconut Flour Cheesy Garlic Biscuits..................138

  16.Radish Chips...139

  17.Flatbread..139

  18.Avocado Fries..140

  19.Pita-Style Chips..141

  20.Roasted Eggplant..141

21.Parmesan-Herb Focaccia Bread 142

22.Quick and Easy Home Fries 143

23.Jicama Fries 144

24.Fried Green Tomatoes 145

25.Fried Pickles 145

26.Pork and Potatoes 146

27.Pork and Fruit Kebabs 147

28.Steak and Vegetable Kebabs....................................... 147

29.Spicy Grilled Steak.. 148

30.Greek Vegetable Skillet 149

31.Light Herbed Meatballs... 149

32.Brown Rice and Beef-Stuffed Bell Peppers 150

33.Beef and Broccoli 151

34.Beef and Fruit Stir-Fry 151

35.Perfect Garlic Butter Steak 152

36.Crispy Pork Medallions 153

37.Parmesan Meatballs 154

38.Tricolor Beef Skewers 155

39.Yogurt Beef Kebabs 156

40.Agave Beef Kebabs 158

41.Beef Skewers with Potato Salad 160

42.Classic Souvlaki Kebobs.. 161

43.Harissa Dipped Beef Skewers 162

44.Onion Pepper Beef Kebobs 163

45.Mayo Spiced Kebobs 164

46.Beef with Orzo Salad.. 165

47.Beef Zucchini Shashliks 167

48.Delicious Zucchini Mix 168

49.Swiss Chard and Sausage 168

50.Swiss Chard Salad...169

51.Spanish Greens 170

52.Flavored Air Fried Tomatoes..............................171

53.Italian Eggplant Stew 172

54.Rutabaga and Cherry Tomatoes Mix.................172

55.Garlic Tomatoes..173

56.Tomato and Basil Tart...174

57.Zucchini Noodles Delight...................................174

58.Simple Tomatoes and Bell Pepper Sauce..........175

59.Salmon with Thyme & Mustard 176

60.Lemon Garlic Fish Fillet 177

61.Blackened Tilapia 178

62.Fish & Sweet Potato Chips..................................178

63.Brussels Sprout Chips 179

64.Shrimp Spring Rolls with Sweet Chili Sauce 180

65.Coconut Shrimp and Apricot 181

66.Coconut Shrimp and Lime Juice........................183

67.Lemon Pepper Shrimp 184

68.Air Fryer Shrimp Bang...185

69.Crispy Nachos Prawns 185

70.Coconut Pumpkin Bars 186

71.Almond Peanut Butter Bars 187

72.Delicious Lemon Bars..188

73.Easy Egg Custard 189

74.Flavors Pumpkin Custard....................................190

75.Almond Butter Cookies..191

76.Tasty Pumpkin Cookies.......................................192

77.Almond Pecan Cookies 192

78.Butter Cookies...194

79.Tasty Brownie Cookies 195

80.Tasty Gingersnap Cookies 195

81.Simple Lemon Pie 196

82.Flavorful Coconut Cake 197

83.Easy Lemon Cheesecake 198

84.Lemon Butter Cake 199

85.Cream Cheese Butter Cake 200

86.Easy Ricotta Cake 201

87.Strawberry Muffins 201

88.Mini Brownie Muffins 202

89.Cinnamon Cheesecake Bars 203

90.Strawberry Cobbler 204

91.Baked Zucchini Fries 205

92.Roasted Heirloom Tomato with Baked Feta 206

93.Garam Masala Beans 207

94.Crisp Potato Wedges 208

95.Crispy Onion Rings 209

96.Cheese Lasagna and Pumpkin Sauce 210

97.Pasta Wraps 211

98.Homemade Tater Tots 212

99.Mushroom, Onion, and Feta Frittata 213

100.Roasted Bell Pepper Vegetable Salad 214

Conclusion 215

The Complete Air Fryer Cookbook

The Ultimate Cookbook With 100 Quick and Delicious Recipes for Quick and Easy Meals

By Marisa Smith

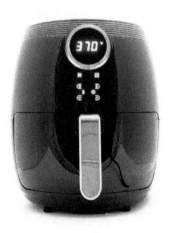

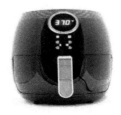

Introduction
Air fryers have seen a major increase in popularity, marketed as a healthy, guilt-free way to eat your favorite fried foods. These are believed to help increase the fat content of popular foods such as burgers, empanadas, chicken wings, and sticks of fish. But how good does an air fryer cook, exactly? The book will look at the facts to determine if many brands of air fryers do not need oil to work with the machine, but the taste of deep-fried food items can be improved by a few teaspoons. While air-fried food can be enjoyed with no oil, the benefit of the air fryer is that it only requires very little quantity.

Air Fryer Recipes

1.Basil Tomato Frittata

Total time: 35 min

Prep time: 15 min

Cook time: 20 min

Yield: 4 servings

Ingredients:

- 12 eggs
- 1/2 cup cheddar cheese, grated
- 1 1/2 cups cherry tomatoes, cut in half
- 1/2 cup fresh basil, chopped
- 1 cup baby spinach, chopped
- 1/2 cup yogurt
- Pepper
- Salt

Directions:

1. Spray with cooking spray on a baking dish and set aside.

2. Wire rack insertion at rack position 6. Pick bake, set temperature to 390 f, 35-minute timer. To preheat the oven, press start.

3. Whisk the eggs and yogurt together in a big bowl.

4. Layer a baking dish of spinach, lettuce, onions, and cheese. Pour the spinach mixture over the egg mixture, with pepper and salt, season.

5. Bake for 35 minutes in the oven.

6. Enjoy and serve.

2.Italian Breakfast Frittata

Total time: 35 min

Prep time: 15 min

Cook time: 20 min

Yield: 4 servings

Ingredients:

- Eight eggs
- 1 tbsp. fresh parsley, chopped
- 3 tbsp. parmesan cheese, grated
- Two small zucchinis, chopped and cooked
- 1/2 cup pancetta, chopped and cooked
- Pepper
- Salt

Directions:

1. Spray with cooking spray on a baking dish and set aside.

2. Wire rack insertion at rack position 6. Pick bake, set temperature to 350 f, 20-minute timer. To preheat the oven, press start.

3. Mix the eggs with pepper and salt in a mixing cup. Stir well and add parsley, cheese, zucchini, and pancetta.

4. Pour the egg mixture into the baking dish that has been prepared.

5. Bake a 20-minute frittata.

6. Enjoy and serve.

3.Healthy Baked Omelets

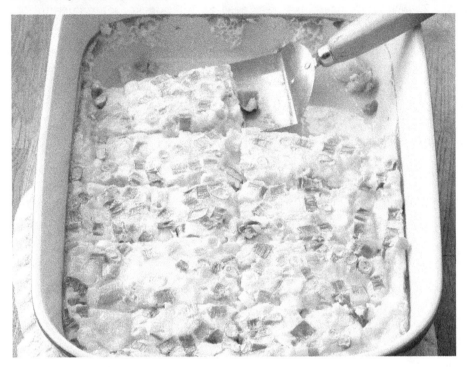

Total time: 45 min

Prep time: 10 minutes

Cooking time: 35 minutes

Yield: 6 servings

Ingredients:

- 8 eggs
- 1 cup bell pepper, chopped
- 1/2 cup onion, chopped
- 1/2 cup cheddar cheese, shredded
- 6 oz. ham, diced and cooked
- 1 cup milk
- Pepper
- Salt

Directions:

1. With cooking sauce, spray an 8-inch baking dish and put it aside.

2. Wire rack insertion at rack position 6. Pick bake, set temperature to 350 f, 45-minute timer. To preheat the oven, press start.

3. In a big cup, mix the milk, pepper, and salt with the eggs. Add the remaining ingredients and stir well.

4. Pour the egg mixture into the baking dish that has been prepared.

5. Bake for 45 minutes for an omelet.

6. Slicing and cooking.

4.Easy Egg Casserole

Total time: 55 min

Prep time: 10 min

Cook time: 45min

Yield: 8 servings

Ingredients:

- 8 eggs
- 1/2 tsp. garlic powder
- 2 cups cheddar cheese, shredded
- 1 cup milk
- 24 oz. frozen hash browns, thawed
- 1/2 onion, diced
- One red pepper, diced
- Four bacon slices, diced
- 1/2 lb. turkey breakfast sausage
- Pepper
- Salt

Directions:

1. Spray a 9*13-inch baking dish with cooking spray and set aside.
2. Insert wire rack in rack position 6. Select bake, set temperature 350 f, timer for 50 minutes. Press start to preheat the oven.
3. Cook breakfast sausage in a pan over medium heat until cooked through. Drain well and set aside.
4. Cook bacon in the same pan. Drain well and set aside.
5. In a mixing bowl, whisk eggs with milk, garlic powder, pepper, and salt. Add 1 cup cheese, hash browns, onion, red pepper, bacon, and sausage and stir well.

6. Pour the entire egg mixture into the baking dish. Sprinkle remaining cheese on top.

7. Cover the dish with foil and bake for 50 minutes. Remove foil and bake for 5 minutes more.

8. Serve and enjoy.

5.Flavor Packed Breakfast Casserole

Total time: 50 min

Prep time: 10 minutes

Cook time: 40 minutes

Yield: 8 servings

Ingredients:

- 1 tsp. garlic powder
- 1 cup milk
- 12 eggs
- 1/2 cup cheddar cheese, shredded
- Two bell pepper, cubed
- 4 small potatoes, cubed
- 2 cups sausage, cooked and diced
- Pepper
- 1/4 cup onion, diced
- Salt

Directions:

1. With cooking oil, spray a 9*13-inch baking dish and put it aside.

2. Wire rack insertion at rack position 6. Pick bake, set temperature to 350 f, 40-minute timer. To preheat the oven, press start.

3. Add the cream, garlic powder, spice, and salt to the eggs in a big cup.

4. To the baking dish, add the bacon, bell peppers, and potatoes. Pour over the sausage mixture with the egg mixture. Sprinkle of onion and cheese.

5. Bake for 40 minutes in a casserole.

6. Slicing and cooking.

6.Vegetable Sausage Egg Bake

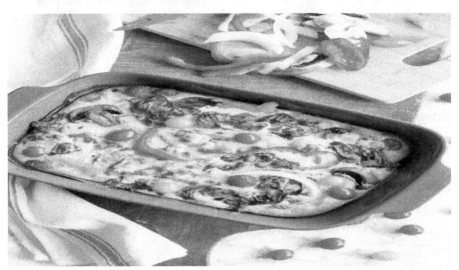

Total time: 45 min

Prep time: 10 minutes

Cook time: 35 minutes

Yield: 4 servings

Ingredients:

- Ten eggs
- 1 cup spinach, diced
- 1/2 cup almond milk
- Pepper
- 1 lb. sausage, cut into 1/2-inch pieces
- 1 cup onion, diced
- 1 cup pepper, diced
- 1 tsp. garlic powder
- Salt

Directions:

23

1. With cooking sauce, spray an 8*8-inch baking dish and put it aside.

2. Wire rack insertion at rack position 6. Pick bake, set temperature to 390 f, 35-minute timer. To preheat the oven, press start.

3. Whisk the eggs in a cup of milk and spices. Attach the sausage and vegetables and stir to mix.

4. Pour the egg mixture into the baking dish that has been prepared. For 35 minutes, roast.

5. Slicing and cooking.

7.Ham Egg Brunch Bake

Preparation time: 10 minutes

Cooking time: 60 minutes

Servings: 6

Ingredients:

- 4 eggs
- 20 oz. hash browns
- One onion, chopped
- 2 cups ham, chopped
- 3 cups cheddar cheese, shredded
- 1 cup sour cream
- 1 cup milk
- Pepper
- Salt

Directions:

1. Spray a 9*13-inch baking dish with cooking spray and set aside.

2. Insert wire rack in rack position 6. Select bake, set temperature 375 f, timer for 35 minutes. Press start to preheat the oven.

3. In a large mixing bowl, whisk eggs with sour cream, milk, pepper, and salt. Add 2 cups cheese and stir well.

4. Cook onion and ham in a medium pan until onion is softened.

5. Add hash brown to the pan and cook for 5 minutes.

6. Add onion ham mixture into the egg mixture and mix well.

7. Pour egg mixture into the prepared baking dish. Cover the dish with foil and bake for 35 minutes.

8. Remove foil and bake for 25 minutes more.

9. Slice and serve.

8.Cheese Broccoli Bake

Total time: 40 min

Prep time: 10 min

Cook time: 30 min

Yield: 12 servings

Ingredients:

- 12 eggs
- 1 1/2 cup cheddar cheese, shredded
- 2 cups broccoli florets, chopped
- 1 small onion, diced
- 1 cup milk
- Pepper
- Salt

Directions:

1. With cooking sauce, spray an 8*8-inch baking dish and put it aside.

2. Wire rack insertion at rack position 6. Pick bake, set temperature to 390 f, 35-minute timer. To preheat the oven, press start.

3. Whisk the eggs in a cup of milk and spices. Attach the sausage and vegetables and stir to mix.

4. Pour the egg mixture into the baking dish that has been prepared. For 35 minutes, roast.

5. Slicing and cooking.

9.   Cheese Ham Omelets

Total time: 35 min

Prep time: 10 min

Cook time: 25 min

Yield: 6 servings

Ingredients:

- 8 eggs
- 1 cup ham, chopped
- 1 cup cheddar cheese, shredded
- 1/3 cup milk
- Pepper
- Salt

Directions:

1. With cooking oil, spray a 9*9-inch baking dish and put it aside.

2. Wire rack insertion at rack position 6. Pick bake, set temperature to 390 f, 25-minute timer. To preheat the oven, press start.

3. In a big cup, mix the milk, pepper, and salt with the eggs. Stir in the cheese and ham.

4. In the prepared baking dish, add in the egg mixture and bake for 25 minutes.

5. Slicing and cooking.

9.Sweet Potato Frittata

Total time: 40 min

Prep time: 10 min

Cook time: 30 min

Yield: 6 servings

Ingredients:

- 10 eggs
- 1/4 cup goat cheese, crumbled
- 1 onion, diced
- 1 sweet potato, diced
- 2 cups broccoli, chopped
- 1 tbsp. olive oil
- Pepper
- Salt

Directions:

1. Spray with cooking spray on a baking dish and set aside.

2. Wire rack insertion at rack position 6. Pick bake, set temperature to 390 f, 20-minute timer. To preheat the oven, press start.

3. Heat oil over medium heat in a pan. Add the sweet potato, broccoli, and onion, then simmer for 10-15 minutes or until tender.

4. Mix the eggs with pepper and salt in a large mixing cup.

5. Cooked vegetables are moved to the baking dish. Pour over the vegetables with the egg mixture. Sprinkle with the goat's cheese and roast for 15-20 minutes.

6. Slicing and serving.

10. Toasty Grilled Chicken with Cauliflower and Garlic Butter

Total time: 45 min

Prep time: 10 min

Cook time: 35 min

Yield: 2 servings

Ingredients:

- Chicken legs
- 2 chicken legs (about 5 oz. each)
- ½ teaspoon garlic powder
- 1 tablespoon coconut oil
- ½ tablespoon Italian seasoning
- ¼ teaspoon salt
- Garlic butter
- 7 tablespoons unsalted butter, softened
- 2 garlic cloves, pressed
- 1 tablespoon fresh mint, finely chopped (optional)
- Salt and ground black pepper, to taste
- 10 oz. Cauliflower

Directions:

1. Mix the coconut oil and seasoning with the chicken wings.

2. For 60 minutes, set the air fryer to 350 degree F. You should flip it if it's 30 minutes out. They used forks and it was so simple.

3. Cut the florets of the cauliflower and cut the stem. Put to a boil in salty water in a saucepan for 5 minutes. To keep it warm, drain the water and put the lid on. Combine all the ingredients: a little bowl of garlic butter. Using cauliflower and garlic butter to serve the chicken.

11. Garlic Turkey

Total time: 30 min

Prep time: 10 min

Cook time: 20 min

Yield: 2 servings

Ingredients:

- 2 tablespoons coconut oil
- 2 lbs. turkey drumsticks
- Salt and pepper
- 1 lime, the juice
- 2 tablespoons avocado oil
- 7 garlic cloves, sliced
- ½ cup fresh basil, finely chopped

Directions:

1. Preheat up to 360 degrees Fahrenheit for your air fryer.
2. In an oil-greased baking pan, put the turkey bits. Salt and pepper with generosity.
3. Drizzle over the turkey bits with lime juice and avocado oil. Sprinkle on top of the garlic and parsley.
4. Air fried for 1 hour at 360 degrees Fahrenheit, spinning every 15 minutes or until the temperature within reaches 165 degrees Fahrenheit.

5.

12.Sweet and Sticky Turkey Wings

Total time: 30 min

Prep time: 10 min

Cook time: 20 min

Yield: 2 servings

Ingredients:

- 1 lb. turkey wings
- ½ teaspoon sea salt
- ¼ cup coconut amino
- ¼ teaspoon ginger minced
- 1teaspoon onion, chopped
- ¼ teaspoon garlic minced
- ¼ teaspoon chili flakes

Directions:

1. Preheat your air fryer to 360 degrees Fahrenheit.

2. Sprinkle fine sea salt on the wings

3. Air fry on 360 degrees Fahrenheit for 1 hour, turning every 15 minutes or until internal temperature has reached a temperature of 165 degrees Fahrenheit.

4. Heat a medium to a large skillet over medium heat, and add the coconut amino.

5. Add the minced ginger, minced garlic, chopped onion, and red pepper flakes (if desired). Once the sauce is simmering, start stirring. Keep stirring at regular intervals and adjust the heat as needed to keep cooking soft.

6. Once the sauce has thickened slightly, place the wings in a large heatproof bowl, and pour the sauce over them. Stir to coat and serve with sauce!

7.

13.Tofu and Cabbage Plate

Total time: 30 min

Prep time: 10 min

Cook time: 20 min

Yield: 2 servings

Ingredients:

- 1 cup tofu
- 7 oz. Fresh green cabbage
- ½ red onion
- 1 tablespoon coconut oil
- ½ cup Greek yogurt
- Salt and pepper

Directions:

1. To further extract excess liquid, push your tofu.
2. Split into squares or small bite-sized bits after pressing the tofu.
3. Bringing the air fryer into the basket.
4. Set the temperature to 370 degrees f. Please turn the air fryer on for 12 minutes.
5. Shred the cabbage and put it on a plate using a sharp knife or a mandolin.
6. Thinly slice the onion and add it to the pan, with the tofu and Greek yogurt added.
7. Drizzle the cabbage with coconut oil and apply some salt and pepper to taste.

14.Thai Fish

Total time: 30 min

Prep time: 10 min

Cook time: 20 min

Yield: 2 servings

Ingredients:

- ½ tablespoon coconut oil
- ¾ lbs. tuna, in pieces
- Salt and pepper
- 2 tablespoons olive oil
- 1 tablespoon green curry paste
- 7 oz. Canned, unsweetened coconut cream
- ½ cup fresh basil, chopped
- 1 lb. broccoli

Directions:

9. Put the pieces of fish into the baking tray. Generously salt and pepper and add a tablespoon of coconut oil to each piece of fish.

10. Combine the coconut cream, curry paste and chopped basil in a small bowl and pour over the fish.

11. Grease the bottom of the air fryer basket and place the fillets in the basket. Cook the steaks at 400 degrees for 10 minutes.

12. Meanwhile, cut the cauliflower into small florets and boil in lightly salted water for a few minutes. Serve with fish.

15.Chicken with Parsnips

Total time: 30 min

Prep time: 10 min

Cooking time: 20 min

Yield: 2 servings

Ingredients:

- 1 lb. chicken thighs or chicken drumsticks
- 1lb parsnips, peeled and cut into 2-3 inch pieces
- ½ tablespoon paprika powder
- Salt and pepper
- ¼ cup coconut oil
- ½ cup Greek yogurt
- ½ teaspoon garlic powder

- ½ teaspoon paprika powder
- Salt and pepper, to taste

Directions:

1. Preheat up to 360 degrees Fahrenheit for your air fryer.

2. In a baking pot, placed the chicken and the parsnips. Sprinkle with flour, paprika powder and pepper. Spray and coat generously with olive oil.

3. Fry the air for 1 hour at 360 degrees Fahrenheit, spinning every 15 minutes or until the temperature within exceeds 165 degrees Fahrenheit.

4. Mix the herb with the yogurt and eat along with the roasted chicken and parsnips.

16.Salmon Salad with Boiled Eggs

Total time: 30 min

Prep time: 10 min

Cook time: 20 min

Yield: 2 servings

Ingredients:

- 4 oz. Cucumber
- 2 spring onion
- 5 oz. Salmon
- ½ orange, zest and juice
- ½ cup Greek yogurt
- 1 teaspoon Dijon mustard
- 4 eggs
- 6 oz. Romaine lettuce
- 4 oz. Cherry tomatoes
- 2 tablespoons coconut oil
- Salt and pepper

Directions:

1. Finely chop the cucumber and the onion for the season. Place the salmon, orange, Greek yogurt and mustard in a medium dish. Remove to blend and season with salt and pepper. Only put aside.

2. In the basket, place the rack supplied with the fryer and place the eggs on the rack. Simply position it at the bottom of the air fryer basket if your air fryer does not have a grill. The temperature should be pressed at 250 and the time set at 15 minutes. Take them out and put them into the cool bathroom water to finish frying while the eggs are fried in the fryer. Break the eggs from the outer shell.

3. Place the salmon and egg mixture on a Romaine lettuce bed. Sprinkle with coconut oil and add the tomatoes. With salt and pepper, season.

17. Tomato Mint Soup

Prep time: 10 Minutes

Cook time: 20 Minutes

Yield: 2 servings

Ingredients:

- Oil for spraying
- ½ lb. red tomatoes cut in half
- 1 small red bell pepper quartered
- 1 small yellow onion quartered
- 1 small carrot chopped
- 4 garlic cloves peeled
- 1.5 cups water
- ½ cup coconut cream
- 4 fresh mint leaves finely chopped
- Grated goat cheese optional

Directions:

1. To keep it from sticking, brush the bottom of the basket with a bit of oil. In the air fryer, add the tomatoes, peppers, onions, carrots, garlic cloves and set to 360 degrees Fahrenheit and fry for 25 minutes.

2. In order to ensure an even roast, inspect the air fryer basket in half and shake it.

3. Place the vegetables in a medium-sized saucepan while the fryer is off, and apply the water to the pan. Let them cook the mixture. Decrease the flame and boil for 5 minutes or so. Mix the soup with the hand blender until finished, or let it cool and mix the soup with a conventional blender.

4. Add the coconut cream and mint. With salt and pepper, season. Goat cheese garnish.

18.Fried Cauliflower Rice

Prep time: 10 Minutes

Cook time: 20 Minutes

Servings: 2

Ingredients:

- 1 medium cauliflower
- 1 tablespoon coconut oil
- 3 spring onions, sliced
- 1 teaspoon smoked paprika
- 1/2 teaspoon ground cumin
- 1/4 teaspoon hot chili powder
- Salt
- Black pepper
- 50 g parmesan cheese, grated

Directions:

1. Remove and cut the cauliflower leaves into florets. Place the bomb in a food processor until it looks like rice.

2. Place the cauliflower rice with a little coconut oil in the air-fryer oven. Cook until lightly browned for 20 minutes, Scrape and apply chives, peppers, and seasonings from the sides of the air fryer cooker.

3. Let it cook for 10 more minutes, then add the cheese and let it cook for 5 more minutes. Re-scrape the sides of the oven and serve it with the ingredients of your choosing.

19.Baked Salmon

Total time: 15 min

Prep time: 05 min

Cook time: 10 min

Yield: 2 servings

Ingredients:

- 2 (6-oz.) Salmon fillets
- Kosher salt
- Freshly ground black pepper
- 2 teaspoons coconut oil
- 1 teaspoon garlic powder
- 1/2 teaspoon basil leaves

Directions:

13. Season the whole salmon with salt and pepper. Mix the coconut oil, garlic and basil in a small bowl. Spread on the salmon and place the salmon in the basket.

14. Set the fryer to 400 ° and cook for 10 minutes.

20.Prosciutto-Wrapped Parmesan Asparagus

Total time: 30 min

Prep time: 10 min

Cook time: 20 min

Yield: 4 servings

Ingredients:

- 1-pound of asparagus
- 12 (0.5-ounce) slices of prosciutto
- 1 tablespoon of coconut oil, melted
- 2 teaspoons of lemon juice
- 1/8 teaspoon of red pepper flakes
- 1/3 cup of grated Parmesan cheese
- 2 tablespoons of salted butter, melted

Directions:

1. On a clean work surface, place an asparagus spear on a slice of prosciutto.

2. Drizzle with lemon juice and coconut oil. Sprinkle the red pepper flakes and parmesan over the asparagus. A roll of prosciutto and an asparagus spear. In the Air Fryer, bring the basket in.

3. Set the temperature to 375 degrees F and set the timer for ten more minutes.

4. Sprinkle a roll of asparagus with butter before feeding. Enjoy!

21.Bacon-Wrapped Jalapeño Poppers

Total time: 30 min

Prep time: 10 min

Cook time: 20 min

Yield: 4 servings

Ingredients:

- 6 jalapeños (about 4" long each)
- 3-ounces of full-Fat: cream cheese
- 1/3 cup of shredded medium Cheddar cheese
- 1/4 teaspoon of garlic powder
- 12slices sugar-free bacon

Directions:

1. Break the tops off the jalapeños and slice down the center lengthwise in two parts. Break the white membrane and pepper seeds with care, using a knife.

2. In a large microwave-safe bowl, put the cream cheese, cheddar, and garlic powder. Remove from the microwave and stir for 30 seconds. Combine the jalapeños with a spoon of cheese.

3. Wrap about half of each jalapeño with a strip of bacon, covering the pepper completely. In the Air Fryer, bring the basket in.

4. Set the temperature to 400 degrees F and change the 12-minute timer.

5. Turn on the peppers halfway into the cooking stage. Serve it hot.

22.Garlic Parmesan Chicken Wings

Total time: 30 min

Prep time: 10 min

Cook time: 20 min

Yield: 4 servings

Ingredients:

- 2 pounds of raw chicken wings
- 1 teaspoon of pink Himalayan salt
- 1/2 teaspoon of garlic powder
- 1 tablespoon of baking powder
- 4 tablespoons of unsalted butter, melted
- 1/3 cup of grated Parmesan cheese
- 1/4 teaspoon of dried parsley

Directions:

1. Place the chicken wings, spice, and 1/2 teaspoon of garlic powder, baking powder, and toss in a large cup. Place the wings in the basket with the Air Fryer.
2. Change the temperature and set the timer to 400°F for 25 minutes.
3. During the cooking cycle, toss the basket two to three times.
4. Combine the sugar, parmesan, and parsley in a shallow dish.
5. Take the wings out of the fryer and put them in a large, clean dish. Over the wings, pour the butter mixture and toss until filled. Serve it hot.

23.Spicy Buffalo Chicken Dip

Total time: 30 min

Prep time: 10 min

Cook time: 20 min

Yield: 4 servings

Ingredients:

- 1 cup of cooked, diced chicken breast
- 8 ounces of full-Fat: cream cheese, softened

- 1/2 cup of buffalo sauce

- 1/3 cup of full-Fat: ranch dressing

- 1/3 cup of chopped pickled jalapeños

- 1 ½ cups of shredded medium Cheddar cheese, divided

- 2 scallions, sliced

Directions:

1. Put the chicken in a spacious bowl. Remove cream cheese, ranch dressing and buffalo sauce. Stir until they are well blended and mostly smooth with the spices. Fold the jalapeños along with 1 cup of Cheddar.

2. In a 4-cup circular baking dish, add the mixture and add the rest of the Cheddar on top. Place the dish in a basket with a hairdryer.

3. Switch the temperature to 350°F and set the timer for 10 minutes.

4. The top will be brown and bubbling until finished. And cut scallions on top. Serve it hot.

24.Bacon Jalapeño Cheese Bread

Total time: 30 min

Prep time: 10 min

Cook time: 20 min

Yield: 8 sticks (2 sticks per servings)

Ingredients:

- 2 cups of shredded mozzarella cheese

- ¼ cup of grated Parmesan cheese

- ¼ cup of chopped pickled jalapeños

- 2 large eggs

- 4 slices of sugar-free bacon, cooked and chopped

Directions:

1. In a wide bowl, combine all ingredients. To suit your Air Fryer basket, trim a piece of parchment.

2. With a bit of sweat, dampen your hands and spread the mixture out into a circle. This will need to be divided into two smaller cheese pieces of bread, depending on the size of your fryer.

3. In the Air Fryer basket, put the parchment and cheese bread.

4. Change the temperature and set the timer to 320°F for 15 minutes.

5. Flip the bread gently while you have 5 minutes left.

6. The top will be golden brown when fully baked. Serve it hot and drink it!

25.Pizza Rolls

Total time: 30 min

Prep time: 10 min

Cook time: 20 min

Yield: 8 sticks (2 sticks per servings)

Ingredients:

- 2 cups of shredded mozzarella cheese
- 1/2 cup of almond flour 2 large eggs
- 72 slices of pepperoni
- 8 (1-ounce) mozzarella string cheese sticks, cut into 3 pieces
- 2 tablespoons of unsalted butter, melted
- 1/4 teaspoon of garlic powder
- ½ teaspoon of dried parsley
- 2 tablespoons of grated Parmesan cheese

Directions:

1. Place the mozzarella and almond flour in a big, microwave-proof dish. 1-minute microwave. Remove the Bowland mix until a ball of dough emerges. If required, microwave for 30 more seconds.

2. Crack the eggs in the bowl and combine until they form a smooth dough ball. With water, wet your hands and knead the dough briefly.

3. Tear off two large pieces of parchment paper and spray non-stick cooking spray on one side of each one.

4. Between the two boards, put the dough ball, with the sprayed sides facing the dough. To stretch the dough out to a thickness of 1/4', use a rolling pin.

5. To slice into 24 rectangles, use a knife. Put 3 pepperoni slices on each rectangle and 1 piece of string cheese.

6. Fold the rectangle in two, covering the filling with pepperoni and cheese. Closed pinch or roll sides. Cut and insert a strip of parchment in the basket to match the Air Fryer basket. Put the parchment on the rolls.

7. Change the temperature and set the timer to 350°F for 10 minutes.

8. Open the fryer after 5 minutes and rotate the rolls of pizza. Restart the fryer and finish frying until the rolls of pizza are golden.

9. Place butter, garlic powder and parsley in a small bowl. Brush the mixture over baked pizza rolls and sprinkle with parmesan. Eat warm. Serve warm.

27.Bacon Cheeseburger Dip

Total time: 30 min

Prep time: 10 min

Cook time: 20 min

Yield: 4 sticks (2 sticks per servings)

Ingredients:

- 8 ounces of full-Fat: cream cheese
- 1/4 cup of full-Fat: mayonnaise
- 1/4 cup of full-Fat: sour cream
- 1/4 cup of chopped onion
- 1 teaspoon of garlic powder
- 1 tablespoon of Worcestershire sauce 1
- 1/4 cups of shredded medium Cheddar cheese, divided
- ½-pound of cooked 80/20 ground beef
- 6 slices of sugar-free bacon, cooked and crumbled
- 2 large pickle spears, chopped.

Directions:

1. In a large microwave-safe bowl, place the cream cheese and microwave for 45 seconds. Stir in mayonnaise, sour cream, onion, powdered garlic, and one cup of Worcestershire Cheddar sauce. Add the bacon and the ground beef. Sprinkle over leftover Cheddar.

2. Place the bowl in 6 "and put it in the basket of the Air Fryer.

3. Set the temperature to 400° F and adjust the timer for 10 minutes.

4. When the top is golden, bubbling sprinkles the pickles over the dish and serves warm.

28.Pork Rind Tortillas

Total time: 30 min

Prep time: 10 min

Cook time: 20 min

Yield: 4 sticks (2 sticks per servings)

Ingredients:

- 1-ounce of pork rinds
- 3/4 cup of shredded mozzarella cheese
- 2 tablespoons of full-Fat: cream cheese
- 1 large egg

Directions:

1. Mount a food processor with pork rinds and pulse until finely soiled.

2. In a big, secure microwave dish, put the mozzarella. Break-in the cream cheese into small pieces and add to the bowl. Microwave for 30 seconds, or before all forms of cheese are melted, and a ball is quickly blended. Apply the ground pork rinds and the egg to the cheese mixture.

3. Continue to stir until a ball shapes the mixture. If it cools too much and the cheese hardens, so microwave for 10 more seconds.

4. Put aside the dough into four little balls. Between two parchment sheets, put each dough ball and roll onto a 1/4 flat mat.

5. Place tortillas in a single layer Air Fryer basket; if necessary, operate in batches.

6. Fix the temperature to 400° F for 5 minutes and set the timer.

7. The tortillas would become crispy and solid when fully baked. Serve and enjoy it immediately!

8.

29.Mozzarella Sticks

Total time: 30 min

Prep time: 10 min

Cook time: 20 min

Yield: 4 sticks (2 sticks per servings)

Ingredients:

- 6 (1-ounce) mozzarella string cheese sticks
- 1/2 cup of grated Parmesan cheese
- ½- an ounce of pork rinds, finely ground
- 1 teaspoon of dried parsley
- 2 large eggs

Directions:

1. Place the mozzarella sticks on a cutting board and cut them in half. Freeze for 45 minutes or until strong, to stand. When freezing overnight, after 1 hour, cut frozen sticks and place them for future use in an airtight zip-top storage container.

2. In a large bowl, combine the parmesan, ground pork rinds, and parsley together.

3. In a medium cup, whisk the eggs together.

4. Place the frozen mozzarella on top of the beaten eggs, then coat with the Parmesan sauce. For discarded pins, repeat. Place the Air Fryer mozzarella sticks in the bowl.

5. For 10 minutes, change the temperature to 400° F and set the timer to golden.

6. Serve it warm and eat it!

30.Bacon-Wrapped Onion Rings

Total time: 30 min

Prep time: 10 min

Cook time: 20 min

Yield: 4 (2 per servings)

Ingredients:

- 1 large onion, peeled
- 1 tablespoon of sriracha
- 8 slices of sugar-free bacon

Directions:

1. Break the ointment into 1/4-inch thick slices. Take two onion slices and bind the bacon around the loops. For the remaining onion and bacon, repeat.

2. Fix the temperature for 10 minutes to 350° F and adjust the timer.

3. To flip the onion rings halfway through the cooking time, use pliers. Once fully cooked, the bacon will be crispy. Eat hot and enjoy it!

31. Crusted Chicken Tenders

Preparation time: 5 minutes

Cooking time: 15 minutes

Servings: 3

Ingredients:

- ½ cup all-purpose flour
- 2 eggs, beaten
- ½ cup seasoned breadcrumbs
- Salt and freshly ground black pepper, to taste
- 2 tablespoons olive oil
- ¾ pound chicken tenders

Directions:

1. Place the flour in a bowl.
2. Place the eggs in a second bowl.
3. Mix the breadcrumbs, salt, black pepper and oil together in a third dish.
4. Cover the chicken bowls with flour,
5. Dip into the eggs and then coat generously with the combination of breadcrumbs.

6. The air fryer should be preheated to 330 degrees F. Arrange the chicken tenderloin in a basket of air fryers. Cook for 10 minutes, roughly.

7. Set the air fryer to 390 degrees f for now.

8. Cook for 5 more minutes or so.

32.Air Fryer Chicken Parmesan

Preparation time: 5 minutes

Cooking time: 9 minutes

Servings: 4

Ingredients:

- ½ c. Keto marinara
- 6 tbsp. Mozzarella cheese
- 1 tbsp. Melted ghee
- 2 tbsp. Grated parmesan cheese
- 6 tbsp. Gluten-free seasoned breadcrumbs
- 8-ounce chicken breasts

Directions:

1. Make sure you preheat the air fryer to 360 degrees. Using olive oil to mist the basket.

2. Mix the parmesan cheese with the breadcrumbs. Just melt ghee.

3. Brush melted the chicken with ghee and dip into the mixture of breadcrumb.

4. In an air fryer, put the coated chicken and cover it with olive oil.

5. Pour into the rack/basket of the oven. Place the rack on the air fryer's center shelf. Set the temperature to 360 degrees F, and set the time for 6 minutes. Cook 2 breasts for 6 minutes and put a tablespoon of sauce and 11/2 tablespoons of mozzarella cheese on top of each breast. Cook for a further three minutes to melt the cheese.

6. As you replicate the procedure with the remaining breasts, keep the cooked parts warm.

33.Chicken Bbq Recipe from Peru

Preparation time: 5 minutes

Cooking time: 40 minutes

Servings: 4

Ingredients:

- ½ teaspoon dried oregano
- 1 teaspoon paprika
- 1/3 cup soy sauce
- 2 ½ pounds chicken, quartered
- 2 tablespoons fresh lime juice
- 2 teaspoons ground cumin
- 5 cloves of garlic, minced

Directions:

15. After placing all the ingredients in a zip-lock bag, keep the marinade in the refrigerator for 2 hours.

16. Preheat the air fryer to 390°f and place the grilling pan in the air fryer.

17. The chicken has to be grilled for 40 minutes and turn sides every 10 minutes while grilling.

34.Ricotta and Parsley Stuffed Turkey Breasts

Preparation time: 5 minutes

Cooking time: 25 minutes

Servings: 4

Ingredients:

- 1 turkey breast, quartered
- 1 cup ricotta cheese
- 1/4 cup fresh Italian parsley, chopped
- 1 teaspoon garlic powder
- 1/2 teaspoon cumin powder
- 1 egg, beaten
- 1 teaspoon paprika
- Salt and ground black pepper, to taste
- Crushed tortilla chips

- 1 ½ tablespoon extra-virgin olive oil

Directions:

1. Firstly, using a rolling pin, flatten out each slice of turkey breast. Let three mixing bowls packed.

2. Combine the parsley, garlic powder, and cumin powder with the ricotta cheese in a small dish.

3. Place the mixture of ricotta/parsley in the middle of each slice. Repeat and roll them up with the remaining bits of the turkey breast.

4. Whisk the egg along with the paprika in another small dish. Combine the salt, pepper, and smashed tortilla chips in the third small dish.

5. Dip each roll into the whisked egg, then roll it over the mixture of tortilla chips.

6. Move the prepared rolls to the basket of an air fryer. Drizzle the olive oil over everything.

7. Cook for 25 minutes at 350 degrees f, operating in batches. If needed, serve soft, garnished with some extra parsley.

35.Cheesy Turkey-Rice with Broccoli

Preparation time: 5 minutes

Cooking time: 40 minutes

Servings: 4

Ingredients:

- 1 cup cooked, chopped turkey meat
- 1 tablespoon and 1-1/2 teaspoons butter, melted
- 1/2 (10 ounces) package frozen broccoli, thawed
- 1/2 (7 ounces) package whole wheat crackers, crushed
- 1/2 cup shredded cheddar cheese
- 1/2 cup uncooked white rice

Directions:

1. In a saucepan, put 2 cups of water to a boil. Add rice to the mixture and cook for 20 minutes. Turn the fire off and set it aside.

2. Lightly oil the air-fryer baking pan with cooking oil. Combine the fried rice, cheese, ham, and broccoli. To combine, toss well.

3. In a small bowl, combine the melted butter and crushed crackers well. Spread uniformly over the rest of the rice.

4. Pour into the rack/basket of the oven. Place the rack on the air fryer's center shelf. Set the temperature to 360 ° f and set the time to 20 minutes for mild browning of the tops.

5. Serve and enjoy.

36.Jerk Chicken Wings

Preparation time: 10 minutes

Cooking time: 16 minutes

Servings: 6

Ingredients:

- 1 tsp. Salt
- ½ c. Red wine vinegar

- 5 tbsp. Lime juice
- 4 chopped scallions
- 1 tbsp. Grated ginger
- 2 tbsp. Brown sugar
- 1 tbsp. Chopped thyme
- 1 tsp. White pepper
- 1 tsp. Cayenne pepper
- 1 tsp. Cinnamon
- 1 tbsp. Allspice
- 1 habanero pepper (seeds/ribs removed and chopped finely)
- 6 chopped garlic cloves
- 2 tbsp. Low-sodium soy sauce
- 2 tbsp. Olive oil
- 4 pounds of chicken wings

Directions:

1. Combine all the ingredients in a dish, bar the wings. Pour the chicken wings into a gallon bag and add them. To marinate, chill for 2-24 hours.

2. Make sure you preheat your air fryer to 390 degrees F.

3. To remove extra liquids, bring chicken wings into a strainer.

4. Pour half of the wings into the basket of your air fryer. Set the temperature to 390 ° f and set the time to 16 minutes and cook for 14-16 minutes to ensure that you shake halfway through the cooking process.

5. Remove the remaining wings and repeat the process

37. Brazilian Mini Turkey Pies

Preparation Time: 5 Minutes

Cooking Time: 10 Minutes

Servings: 8

Prep + Cook Time: 15 minutes | Servings: 8

Ingredients:

- 1 oz. turkey stock
- 2 oz. whole milk
- 2 oz. coconut milk
- 8 oz. homemade tomato sauce
- 1 tsp. oregano
- 1 tbsp. coriander
- Salt and ground black pepper to taste
- 2 oz. turkey, cooked and shredded
- Flour
- 8 slices filo pastry
- 1 small egg beaten

Directions:

1. Get a clean mixing bowl and put all your wet ingredients, except the egg. Mix well.

2. The result should be a pale-looking sauce – the stock for your pie. Now add the seasoning and turkey before mixing again. Finally, set the mixture aside.

3. To each of your little pie cases, line them with a bit of flour before the filo pastry. This prevents them from sticking. Each pie should use up one sheet of filo, and it should be centrally positioned such that you can easily fold over the extra pastry for the top of the pie.

4. Add the mixture to every mini pie pot until they are ¾ full.

5. Cover the top with the remaining pastry before brushing the egg along the top.

6. Transfer the mini pie pot into the air fryer, set the temperature to 360 F and allow to cook for 10 minutes.

7. Serve

38.Pork Taquitos

Preparation time: 10 minutes

Cooking time: 16 minutes

Servings: 8

Ingredients:

- 1 juiced lime
- 10 whole-wheat tortillas
- 2 ½ c. Shredded mozzarella cheese
- 30 ounces of cooked and shredded pork tenderloin

Directions:

1. Make sure to preheat your air fryer to 380 degrees F.

2. Drizzle pork with lime juice and gently mix.

3. Using a dampened paper towel to smooth the tortillas in the oven.

4. Apply to each tortilla roughly 3 ounces of pork and 1/4 cup of shredded cheese. Wrap them up securely.

5. Spray a little bit of olive oil on the air fryer basket.

6. Set the temperature to 380 degrees F, and set the time for 10 minutes. 7-10 minutes before tortillas turn a faint golden color, make sure to rotate halfway through the cooking process and then enjoy

39.Panko-breaded pork chops

Preparation time: 5 minutes

Cooking time: 12 minutes

Servings: 6

Ingredients:

- 5 (3½- to 5-ounce) pork chops (bone-in or boneless)
- Seasoning salt
- Pepper

- ¼ cup all-purpose flour
- 2 tablespoons panko bread crumbs
- Cooking oil

Directions:

18. Season the pork chops with the seasoning salt and pepper to taste.

19. Sprinkle the flour on both sides of the pork chops, then coat both sides with panko bread crumbs.

20. Place the pork chops in the air fryer. Stacking them is okay.

21. Spray the pork chops with cooking oil. Pour into the oven rack/basket. Place the rack on the middle shelf of the air fryer. Set temperature to 375°f, and set time to 6 minutes. Cook for 6 minutes.

22. Open the air fryer and flip the pork chops. Cook for an additional 6 minutes

23. Cool before serving.

24. Typically, bone-in pork chops are juicier than boneless. If you prefer really juicy pork chops, use bone-in.

40. Apricot glazed pork tenderloins

Preparation time: 5 minutes

Cooking time: 30 minutes

Servings: 3

Ingredients:

- 1 teaspoon salt
- 1/2 teaspoon pepper
- 1-lb pork tenderloin
- 2 tablespoons minced fresh rosemary or 1 tablespoon dried rosemary, crushed
- 2 tablespoons olive oil, divided
- Garlic cloves, minced
- Apricot glaze ingredients:
- 1 cup apricot preserves
- Garlic cloves, minced

- 4 tablespoons lemon juice

Directions:

1. Brush the seasoning or well-mixed seasoning of salt, pepper, garlic and olive oil pork. Pork can be cut into two halves to fit into an air fryer if required.

2. Use cooking spray to grease the air fryer pan and place the port onto it.

3. Cook each side of pork in a preheated 390°f air fryer for 3 minutes.

4. Mix well all of the glaze ingredients in a small bowl.

5. Cook at 330°f for 20 minutes.

6. Serve and enjoy.

41.Barbecue Flavored Pork Ribs

Preparation time: 5 minutes

Cooking time: 15 minutes

Servings: 6

Ingredients:

- ¼ cup honey, divided
- ¾ cup bbq sauce
- 2 tablespoons tomato ketchup
- 1 tablespoon Worcestershire sauce
- 1 tablespoon soy sauce
- ½ teaspoon garlic powder
- Freshly ground white pepper, to taste
- 1¾ pound pork ribs

Directions:

1. In a large bowl, mix together 3 tablespoons of honey and the remaining ingredients except for pork ribs.

2. Refrigerate to marinate for about 20 minutes.

3. Preheat the air fryer to 355 degrees f.

4. Place the ribs in an air fryer basket.

5. Cook for about 13 minutes.

6.   Remove the ribs from the air fryer and coat with the remaining honey.

7.   Serve hot.

42.Balsamic Glazed Pork Chops

Preparation time: 5 minutes

Cooking time: 50 minutes

Servings: 4

Ingredients:

- ¾ cup balsamic vinegar
- 1 ½ tablespoons sugar
- 1 tablespoon butter
- 3 tablespoons olive oil
- Tablespoons salt
- 3 pork rib chops

Directions:

1.   Place all ingredients in a bowl and allow the meat to marinate in the fridge for at least 2 hours.

2.   Preheat the air fryer to 390°f.

3.   Place the grill pan accessory in the air fryer.

4.   Grill the pork chops for 20 minutes, making sure to flip the meat every 10 minutes for even grilling.

5.   Meanwhile, pour the balsamic vinegar on a saucepan and allow to simmer for at least 10 minutes until the sauce thickens.

6.   Brush the meat with the glaze before serving.

43.Rustic Pork Ribs

Preparation time: 5 minutes

Cooking time: 15 minutes

Servings: 4

Ingredients:

- 1 rack of pork ribs
- 3 tablespoons dry red wine

- 1 tablespoon soy sauce

- 1/2 teaspoon dried thyme

- 1/2 teaspoon onion powder

- 1/2 teaspoon garlic powder

- 1/2 teaspoon ground black pepper

- 1 teaspoon smoked salt

- 1 tablespoon cornstarch

- 1/2 teaspoon olive oil

Directions:

1. First, preheat your air fryer to 390 degrees f. Marinate after mixing all the ingredients for at least 1 hour.

2. Set temperature to 390°f, for 25 minutes and place the rack on the middle shelf of the air fryer. Cook the ribs for almost 25 minutes.

3. Serve hot.

44.Keto Parmesan Crusted Pork Chops

Preparation time: 10 minutes

Cooking time: 15 minutes

Servings: 8

Ingredients:

- 3 tbsp. Grated parmesan cheese

- 1 c. Pork rind crumbs

- 2 beaten eggs

- ¼ tsp. Chili powder

- ½ tsp. Onion powder

- 1 tsp. Smoked paprika

- ¼ tsp. Pepper

- ½ tsp. Salt

- 4-6 thick boneless pork chops

Directions:

1. Preheat your air fryer to 400 degrees F.

2. Season all sides of the pork chops with pepper and salt.

3. Pulse pork rinds into crumbs in a food processor. And other seasonings, combine the crumbs.

4. Whip the eggs and add them to another bowl.

5. Dip pork chops into eggs and then into a combination of pork rind crumbs.

6. Spray the olive oil on an air fryer and add the pork chops to the basket. Set the temperature to 400 degrees F, and set the time for 15 minutes.

45.Crispy Fried Pork Chops the Southern Way

Preparation time: 10 minutes

Cooking time: 25 minutes

Servings: 4

Ingredients:

- ½ cup all-purpose flour
- ½ cup low-fat buttermilk
- ½ teaspoon black pepper
- ½ teaspoon tabasco sauce
- Teaspoon paprika
- 3 bone-in pork chops

Directions:

1. In a zip-lock bag, put the buttermilk and the hot sauce and add the pork chops. Enable it to marinate in the fridge for at least an hour.

2. Combine the rice, paprika, and black pepper in a dish.

3. Let the pork out of the zip-lock container and dredge it with the flour mixture.

4. Preheat to 390°f with the air fryer.

5. With cooking oil, brush the pork chops.

6. Pour into the rack/basket of the oven. Place the rack on the air fryer's center shelf. Set the temperature to 390 degrees F, and set the time for 25 minutes.

46.Scrumptious Rib-Eye Steak

Preparation time: 5 minutes

Cooking time: 15 minutes

Servings: 2

Ingredients:

- 2 rib-eye steaks, sliced 1 1/2- inch pieces
- 1/2 cup soy sauce
- 1/4 cup olive oil
- 4 teaspoons grill seasoning

Directions:

1. Combine the steaks, salt, olive oil and soy sauce in a resealable bag; shake to cover well and allow to marinate for at least 2 hours.

2. Pick the meat and discard the marinade from the bag.

3. The air fryer toast oven pan is added with a splash of water and then preheated to 400 degrees.

4. In the basket, add the meat and simmer for 7 minutes. Switch the steak over and cook for an extra 8 minutes. Remove the meat and leave to rest before serving for at least 5 minutes.

47.Air Fryer Toast Oven Sticky Pork Ribs

Preparation time: 2-12 hours

Cooking time: 15 minutes

Servings: 4

Ingredients:

- 1 rack pork baby back ribs
- 1 tbsp. Oyster sauce
- 2 tbsp. Light soy sauce
- 1 tsp. Dark soy sauce
- 1 tbsp. Mustard
- 1 ½ tbsp. Pure honey
- 5 cloves garlic, halved

- 1-inch fresh garlic, sliced
- For the sauce:
- 1 tbsp. Soy sauce
- 1 tbsp. Fish sauce
- 2 tsp. Toasted rice powder
- 1 tsp. Sugar
- 2 tsp. Red chili flakes
- Freshly squeezed juice of ½ a lemon
- 2 tsp. Finely chopped cilantro
- 1 clove garlic, finely chopped

Directions:

1. To make the marinade, mix all the ingredients for the ribs in a dish, apart from the ribs.
2. Separate the ribs and put the marinade in a wide bowl over the ribs, ensuring that the ribs are well protected. Cover with adhesive tape and marinate for at least 2 hours. Marinate overnight for better results.
3. Set 360 degrees f for your air fryer toast oven,
4. In the air-fryer toast oven, add the ribs, garlic and ginger bits. Do not stir in the juices. Six minutes to prepare, shake well and 6 more minutes to cook.
5. Create the dip by adding all the sauce ingredients while the ribs cook: then set it aside in a small dish.
6. With the dipping sauce, relish the ribs.
7. Enjoy!

48.Coriander Lamb with Pesto' N Mint Dip

Preparation time: 5 minutes

Cooking time: 15 minutes

Servings: 4

Ingredients:

- 1 1/2 teaspoons coriander seeds, ground in a spice mill or mortar with a pestle

- 1 large red bell pepper, cut into 1-inch squares

- 1 small red onion, cut into 1-inch squares

- 1 tablespoon extra-virgin olive oil plus additional for brushing

- 1 teaspoon coarse kosher salt

- 1-pound trimmed lamb meat, cut into 1 1/4-inch cube

- 4 large garlic cloves, minced

- Mint-pesto dip ingredients:

- 1 cup (packed) fresh mint leaves

- 2 tablespoons pine nuts

- 2 tablespoons freshly grated parmesan cheese

- 1 tablespoon fresh lemon juice

- 1 medium garlic clove, peeled

- 1/2 cup (packed) fresh cilantro leaves

- 1/2 teaspoon coarse kosher salt

- 1/2 cup (or more) extra-virgin olive oil

Directions:

1. Puree all the dip ingredients in the blender until smooth and fluffy. Transfer and set aside in a bowl.

2. Mix the coriander, salt, garlic, and oil in a wide cup. Add lamb, toss to cover well. Marinate in the ref for a minimum of an hour.

3. In a skewer, thread the lamb, bell pepper, and onion alternately. Repeat until all ingredients are complete: re-use. Place it in the air fryer on the skewer rack.

4. Cook on 390 halfway through cooking time, turnover, for 8 minutes,

5. Serve on the side and eat with sauce.

49.Cumin-Sichuan Lamb Bbq with Dip

Preparation time: 10 minutes

Cooking time: 25 minutes

Servings: 4

Ingredients:

- 1 1/4 pounds boneless lamb shoulder, cut into 1-inch pieces
- 1 tablespoon Sichuan peppercorns or 1 teaspoon black peppercorns
- 1 teaspoon sugar
- 2 tablespoons cumin seeds
- 2 teaspoons caraway seeds
- 2 teaspoons crushed red pepper flakes
- Finely grated lemon zest (for serving)
- Kosher salt, freshly cracked pepper
- For the garlic yogurt dip:
- 1 garlic clove, grated
- 1 tablespoon fresh lemon juice
- 1 cup plain greek yogurt
- Kosher salt, freshly ground pepper
- 1/2 teaspoon finely grated lemon zest

Directions:

1. Process the cumin seeds, peppercorns, caraway seeds, pepper flakes and sugar in a food processor until smooth.
2. Thread bits of lamb into skewers. With salt, season. Rub the paste all over the bits of meat.
3. Place the rack on the skewer.
4. Cook at 390 or to the optimal density for 5 minutes.
5. Meanwhile, whisk the ingredients well in a medium bowl and set aside.

6. Serve with dip and enjoy.

50.Garlic Lemon-Wine on Lamb Steak

Preparation time: 20 minutes

Cooking time: 1 hour and 30 minutes

Servings: 4

Ingredients:

- ¼ cup extra virgin olive oil
- ½ cup dry white wine
- 1 tablespoon brown sugar
- 2 pounds lamb steak, pounded
- 2 tablespoons lemon juice
- 3 tablespoons ancho chili powder
- 8 cloves of garlic, minced
- Salt and pepper to taste

Directions:

1. Place all the ingredients in a bowl and let the meat marinate for at least 2 hours in the refrigerator.
2. To 390f, preheat the air fryer.
3. Place the accessory for the grill pan in the air-fryer.
4. For 20 minutes per batch, grill the beef.
5. Meanwhile, in a saucepan, pour the marinade and let it boil for 10 minutes before the sauce thickens.

51.Garlic-Rosemary Lamb Bbq

Preparation time: 5 minutes

Cooking time: 12 minutes

Servings: 2

Ingredients:

- 1-lb cubed lamb leg
- Juice of 1 lemon
- Fresh rosemary

- 3 smashed garlic cloves
- Salt and pepper
- 1/2 cup olive oil

Directions:

1. Mix all the ingredients in a shallow bowl, and marinate for 3 hours.
2. Thread bits of lamb into skewers. Place it in an air fryer on a skewer rack.
3. Cook at 390F for 12 minutes. Turnover skewers, halfway through cooking time. Cook in batches if needed.
4. Enjoy and serve.

52.Maras Pepper Lamb Kebab Recipe from Turkey

Preparation time: 5 minutes

Cooking time: 15 minutes

Servings: 2

Ingredients:

- 1-lb lamb meat, cut into 2-inch cubes
- Kosher salt
- Freshly cracked black pepper
- 2 tablespoons maras pepper, or 2 teaspoons other dried chili powder mixed with 1 tablespoon paprika
- 1 teaspoon minced garlic
- 2 tablespoons roughly chopped fresh mint
- 1/2 cup extra-virgin olive oil, divided
- 1/2 cup dried apricots, cut into medium dice

Directions:

1. Combine the pepper, salt, and half of the olive oil in a cup. To coat, add lamb and toss well. Thread out 4 skewers of lamb.
2. Cook at 390 or to the optimal density for 5 minutes.
3. Mix well the remaining oil, mint, garlic, maras pepper, and apricots in a wide bowl. Add the lamb roasted. With salt and pepper, season. Toss well, coat,

4. Enjoy and serve.

53.Saffron Spiced Rack of Lamb

Preparation time: 20 minutes

Cooking time: 1 hour and 10 minutes

Servings: 4

Ingredients:

- ½ teaspoon crumbled saffron threads
- 1 cup plain greek yogurt
- 1 teaspoon lemon zest
- 2 cloves of garlic, minced
- 2 racks of lamb, rib bones frenched
- 2 tablespoons olive oil
- Salt and pepper to taste

Directions:

1. To 390f, preheat the air fryer.
2. Place the accessory for the grill pan in the air-fryer.
3. With salt and pepper to taste, season the lamb meat. Only set aside.
4. Combine the remaining ingredients in a dish.
5. Brush the mixture onto the lamb.
6. Set aside and cook for 1 hour and 10 minutes on the grill pan.

54.Shepherd's Pie Made Of Ground Lamb

Preparation time: 20 minutes

Cooking time: 50 minutes

Servings: 4

Ingredients:

- 1-pound lean ground lamb
- 2 tablespoons and 2 teaspoons all-purpose flour
- Salt and ground black pepper to taste
- 1 teaspoon minced fresh rosemary

- 2 tablespoons cream cheese
- 2 ounces Irish cheese (such as dubliner®), shredded
- Salt and ground black pepper to taste
- 1 tablespoon milk
- 1-1/2 teaspoons olive oil
- 1-1/2 teaspoons butter
- 1/2 onion, diced
- 1/2 teaspoon paprika
- 1-1/2 teaspoons ketchup
- 1-1/2 cloves garlic, minced
- 1/2 (12 ounces) package frozen peas and carrots, thawed
- 1-1/2 teaspoons butter
- 1/2 pinch ground cayenne pepper
- 1/2 egg yolk
- 1-1/4 cups water, or as needed
- 1-1/4 pounds Yukon gold potatoes, peeled and halved
- 1/8 teaspoon ground cinnamon

Directions:

1. Boil a big saucepan of salted water and add the potatoes. Simmer until tender, for 15 minutes.

2. Meanwhile, gently grease the air-fryer baking pan with butter. Melt at 360f for 2 minutes.

3. Mix ground lamb and onion. Cook for 10 minutes, halfway through cooking time, stirring and crumbling.

4. Garlic, ketchup, cinnamon, paprika, black pepper, rosemary, salt, and flour are added. Mix thoroughly and cook for 3 minutes.

5. Add water and pan deglaze. For 6 minutes, continue cooking.

6. Stir in the peas and carrots. Spread the mixture uniformly in the pan.

7. Drain well once the potatoes are finished and move the potatoes to a bowl. Mash the potatoes and stir in the cream cheese, cayenne

pepper, butter and Irish cheese. Mix thoroughly. To taste, season with pepper and salt.

8. Whisk the milk and egg yolk well in a small cup. Stir the mashed potatoes in.

9. Top the mixture of ground lamb with mashed potatoes.

10. Cook for an additional 15 minutes or until the potato tops are lightly browned.

11. Enjoy and serve.

55.Simple Lamb Bbq with Herbed Salt

Preparation time: 20 minutes

Cooking time: 1 hour 20 minutes

Servings: 8

Ingredients:

- 2 ½ tablespoons herb salt

- 2 tablespoons olive oil

- 4 pounds boneless leg of lamb, cut into 2-inch chunks

Directions:

1. Preheat the air fryer to 390 f.

2. Place the grill pan accessory in the air fryer.

3. Season the meat with the herb salt and brush with olive oil.

4. Grill the meat for 20 minutes per batch.

5. Make sure to flip the meat every 10 minutes for even cooking.

56.Greek Lamb Meatballs

Preparation time: 12 minutes

Cooking time: 12 minutes

Servings: 12

Ingredients:

- 1 pound ground lamb

- ½ cup breadcrumbs

- ¼ cup milk
- 2 egg yolks
- 1 teaspoon ground coriander
- 1 teaspoon ground cumin
- 3 garlic cloves, minced
- 1 teaspoon dried oregano
- ½ teaspoon salt
- ½ teaspoon black pepper
- 1 lemon, juiced and zested
- ¼ cup fresh parsley, chopped
- ½ cup crumbled feta cheese
- Olive oil, for shaping
- Tzatziki, for dipping

Directions:

1. Combine all ingredients except olive oil in a large mixing bowl and mix well.

2. Form 12 meatballs, about 2 ounces each. Use olive oil on your hands, so they don't stick to the meatballs. Set aside.

3. Select the broil function on the cosori air fryer toaster oven, set the time to 12 minutes, then press the start/cancel to preheat.

4. Place the meatballs on the food tray, then insert the tray at the top position in the preheated air fryer toaster oven. Press start/cancel.

5. Take out the meatballs when done and serve with a side of tzatziki.

57.Lamb Gyro

Preparation time: 10 minutes

Cooking time: 25 minutes

Servings: 4

Ingredients:

- 1 pound ground lamb

- Tzatziki sauce, to taste
- ¼ red onion, minced
- ¼ cup mint, minced
- ½ teaspoon black pepper
- 12 mint leaves, minced
- 4 slices of pita bread
- ¾ cup hummus
- 1 cup romaine lettuce, shredded
- ½ onion sliced
- 2 cloves garlic, minced
- ½ teaspoon salt
- 1 Roma tomato, diced
- ½ cucumber, skinned and thinly sliced
- ¼ cup parsley, minced
- ⅛ teaspoon rosemary

Directions:

1. Mix ground lamb, red onion, mint, parsley, garlic, salt, rosemary, and black pepper until fully combined.

2. Select the broil function on the cosori air fryer toaster oven, set time to 25 minutes and temperature to 450°f, then press the start/cancel to preheat.

3. Line the food tray with parchment paper and place the ground lamb on top, shaping it into a patty 1-inch-thick and 6 inches in diameter.

4. Insert the food tray at the top position in the preheated air fryer toaster oven, then press the start/cancel.

5. Remove when done and cut into thin slices.

6. Assemble each gyro starting with pita bread, then hummus, lamb meat, lettuce, onion, tomato, cucumber, and mint leaves, drizzle with tzatziki.

7. Serve immediately.

58.Masala Galette

Total time: 30 min

Prep time: 10 min

Cook time: 25 min

Yield: 2 servings

Ingredients:

- 2 tbsp. of garam masala
- 2 medium potatoes boiled and mashed
- 1 ½ cup of coarsely crushed peanuts
- 3 tsp. of ginger finely chopped
- 1-2 tbsp. of fresh coriander leaves
- 2 or 3 green chilies finely chopped
- 1 ½ tbsp. of lemon juice
- Salt and pepper to taste

Directions:

1. Blend into a clean container with the ingredients.
2. Shape this mixture into galettes that are smooth and round.
3. Wet the galettes softly with sweat. Fill each galette with crushed peanuts.
4. Preheat the Air Fryer, at 160° Fahrenheit, for 5 minutes. Place your basket galettes and let them steam at the bottom for another 25 minutes.
5. At the same temperature, just. Go turn them over to cook them. Using ketchup or mint chutney to serve.

59.Potato Samosa

Total time:30 min

Prep time: 10 min

Cook time:20 min

Yield:6 servings

Ingredients:

For wrappers:

- 2 tbsp. of unsalted butter
- 1 ½ cup of all-purpose flour
- A pinch of salt to taste
- Add as much water as required to make the dough stiff and firm

For filling:

- 2-3 big potatoes boiled and mashed
- ¼ cup of boiled peas
- 1 tsp. of powdered ginger
- 1 or 2 green chilies that are finely chopped or mashed
- ½ tsp. of cumin
- 1 tsp. of coarsely crushed coriander
- 1 dry red chili broken into pieces
- A small amount of salt (to the taste)
- ½ tsp. of dried mango powder
- ½ tsp. of red chili powder.
- 1-2 tbsp. Of coriander.

Directions:

1. To keep it stiff to smooth for external wrapping, rub the dough. When the filling is finished, let it rest in a pot.

2. In a saucepan, heat the ingredients and combine well to make a sticky paste. Write the bread out.

3. Cover and flatten the dough into cubes. Break them in half and add the filling afterward. To support you, fold the rims to make a cone shape, use water.

4. For around 5-6 minutes, preheat the Air Fryer at 300 Fahrenheit. Put all the samosas in the basket and shut the basket properly. Hold the Air Fryer, at 200°, for another 20 to 25 minutes.

5. At the halfway point, open the basket, and turn the samosas over for regular preparation. Fry at 250 ° for around 10 minutes after this, to give them the ideal golden-brown shade. Wet to serve. Recommended sides have tamarind or mint chutney.

6.

60.Vegetable Kebab

Total time: 30 min

Prep time: 10 min

Cook time: 20 min

Yield: 2 servings

Ingredients:

- 2 cups of mixed vegetables
- 3 onions chopped
- 5 green chilies-roughly chopped
- 1 ½ tbsp. of ginger paste
- 1 ½ tsp. of garlic paste
- 1 ½ tsp. of salt
- 3 tsp. of lemon juice
- 2 tsp. of garam masala
- 4 tbsp. of chopped coriander
- 3 tbsp. of cream
- 3 tbsp. of chopped capsicum
- 3 eggs
- 2 ½ tbsp. of white sesame seeds

Directions:

1. Grind the ingredients, except for the egg, and make a smooth paste. Coat the paste goods with the mask. Now, pound the eggs and add more salt to them.

2. Scatter the coated vegetables in the egg mixture, then transfer to the sesame seeds and garnish well with herbs. Place them on a stick with the vegetables.

3. Pre-fire the Air Fryer at 160 ° Fahrenheit for roughly 5 minutes. Place the sticks in the basket and simmer for 25 more minutes.

4. Move the clamps to the cook's suite during the cooking process, only at the same temperature.

61.Sago Galette

Total time: 25 min

Prep time: 10 min

Cook time: 25 min

Yield: 2 servings

Ingredients:

- 2 cups of sago soaked
- 1 ½ cup of coarsely crushed peanuts
- 3 tsp. of ginger finely chopped
- 1-2 tbsp. of fresh coriander leaves
- 2 or 3 green chilies finely chopped
- 1 ½ tbsp. of lemon juice
- Salt and pepper to the taste

Directions:

1. Wash the soaked sago with the other ingredients, and place it in a clean tub. Shape this mixture into flat and round galettes.

2. Wet the galettes softly with sweat. Fill each galette with crushed peanuts.

3. Preheat the Air Fryer, at 160° Fahrenheit, for 5 minutes. Place your fry basket galettes and allow them to steam at the bottom, just the same temperature for another 25 minutes. Go to fry and turn them over. Serve with chutney, basil or ketchup.

62.Stuffed Capsicum Baskets

Total time: 25 min

Prep time: 10 min

Cook time: 25 min

Yield: 2 servings

Ingredients:

For baskets:

- 3-4 long capsicum
- ½ tsp. of salt
- ½ tsp. of pepper powder

For filling:

- 1 medium onion finely chopped
- 1 green chili finely chopped
- 2 or 3 large potatoes boiled and mashed
- 1 ½ tbsp. of chopped coriander leaves
- 1 tsp. of fenugreek
- 1 tsp. of dried mango powder
- 1 tsp. of cumin powder
- Salt and pepper to the taste

For topping:

- 3 tbsp. of grated cheese
- 1 tsp. of red chili flakes
- ½ tsp. of oregano
- ½ tsp. of basil
- ½ tsp. of parsley

Directions:

1. Take all the ingredients under the heading "Filling." and put them together in a pan.
2. Cut off the stem of the capsicum. Break out the caps. Remove the seeds as well.
3. Sprinkle over the capsicum inside with some salt and pepper. Switch on, until some time ago, and they were apart.
4. Now fill the intended filling with the hollowed-out capsicums. Sprinkle with the grated cheese, and still add the seasoning.
5. Preheat at 140 ° Fahrenheit for 5 minutes with the Air Fryer. Place the capsicums in and around the basket of fried rice. Let them cook 20 more minutes more temperature, as well. Turn them to hide from cooking in between.

63.Baked Macaroni Pasta

Total time: 25 min

Prep time: 10 min

Cook time: 25 min

Yield: 2 servings

Ingredients:

- 1 cup of pasta
- 7 cups of boiling water
- 1 ½ tbsp. of olive oil
- A pinch of salt

For tossing pasta:

- 1 ½ tbsp. of olive oil
- ½ cup of small carrot pieces
- Salt and pepper to the taste
- ½ tsp. of oregano
- ½ tsp. of basil

For the white sauce:

- 2 tbsp. of olive oil
- 2 tbsp. of all-purpose flour
- 2 cups of milk
- 1 tsp. of dried oregano
- ½ tsp. of dried basil
- ½ tsp. of dried parsley
- Salt and pepper to the taste

Directions:

- Cook the pasta and sieve when finished. Toss the pasta with the ingredients mentioned above and set aside. For the sauce, add the ingredients to a skillet and bring them to a boil.

- To produce a thicker sauce, drop the sauce and begin to boil. Connect the pasta to the sauce and put it in a glass dish garnished with cheese.

- Preheat the Air Fryer, at 160°, for 5 minutes. Place the basket in the bowl and fasten it. Let it proceed to boil for 10 minutes at the same temperature. Hold the sauce, stirring.

64.Macaroni Samosa

Total time: 30 min

Prep time: 10 min

Cook time: 10 min

Yield: 2 servings

Ingredients:

For wrappers:

- 1 cup of all-purpose flour
- 2 tbsp. of unsalted butter
- A pinch of salt to the taste
- Take the amount of water sufficient enough to make a stiff dough

For filling:

- 3 cups of boiled macaroni
- 2 onion sliced
- 2 capsicum sliced
- 2 carrot sliced
- 2 cabbage sliced
- 2 tbsp. of soya sauce
- 2 tsp. of vinegar
- 2 tbsp. of ginger finely chopped
- 2 tbsp. of garlic finely chopped
- 2 tbsp. of green chilies finely chopped
- 2 tbsp. of ginger-garlic paste
- Some salt and pepper to taste
- 2 tbsp. of olive oil
- ½ tsp. of Ajinomoto

Directions:

1. To keep it stiff to smooth for external wrapping, rub the dough. When the filling is full, set the remainder aside in a bowl.

2. In a saucepan, heat the ingredients and combine well to make a sticky paste. Let the color work out.

3. Cover and flatten the dough into cubes. Halve the break-in, then add the filling. To support you, fold the rims to make a cone shape, use water.

4. For around 5-6 minutes, preheat the Air Fryer at 300 Fahrenheit. Place all the samosas in one place, then lock the basket properly. Hold the Air Fryer, at 200°, for another 20 to 25 minutes.

5. Open the bowl and turn over the samosas to cook them uniformly. Afterward, fry at 250 ° for about 10 minutes to give them the perfect golden tan shade. Wet to serve. Tamarinds or green chutney includes the recommended sides.

65.Burritos

Total time: 35 min

Prep time: 10 min

Cook time: 15 min

Yield: 2 servings

Ingredients:

Refried beans:

- ½ cup of red kidney beans (soaked overnight)
- ½ small onion chopped
- 1 tbsp. of olive oil
- 2 tbsp. of tomato puree
- ¼ tsp. of red chili powder
- 1 tsp. of salt to the taste
- 4-5 flour tortillas

Vegetable Filling:

- 1 tbsp. of olive oil
- 1 medium onion finely sliced

- 3 flakes of garlic crushed

- ½ cup of French beans (Slice them lengthwise into thin and long slices)

- ½ cup of mushrooms thinly sliced

- 1 cup of cottage cheese cut in too long and slightly thick fingers

- ½ cup of shredded cabbage

- 1 tbsp. of coriander, chopped

- 1 tbsp. of vinegar

- 1 tsp. of white wine

- A pinch of salt to the taste

- ½ tsp. of red chili flakes

- 1 tsp. of freshly ground peppercorns

- ½ cup of pickled jalapenos (Chop them up finely)

- 2 carrots (Cut into long thin slices)

Salad:

- 1-2 lettuce leaves shredded.

- 1 or 2 spring onions chopped finely. Also, cut the greens.

- 1 tomato. Remove the seeds and chop them into small pieces.

- 1 green chili chopped.

- 1 cup of cheddar cheese, grated.

Directions:

1. Cook the beans along with the onion and garlic and mash them finely. Now, prepare the burrito sauce you're going to need. Make sure you make a sauce that is slightly thick.

2. You may need to cook the ingredients well in a pan for the filling and to ensure that the vegetables on the outside are browned.

3. Place the tortilla and apply a layer of salsa, followed by the beans and the filling in the middle. To make the salad, toss the ingredients together. You'll need to put the salad on top of the filling before rolling it out.

4. At 200 Fahrenheit, preheat the Air Fryer for about 5 minutes. Keep the burritos inside and open the fry basket. Cover the basket

accordingly. For another 15 minutes or so, let the Air Fryer sit at 200 Fahrenheit.

5. Remove the basket and turn all the burritos over halfway through, and get a uniform chef.

66.Cheese and Bean Enchiladas

Total time: 35 min

Prep time: 10 min

Cook time: 15 min

Yield: 2 servings

Ingredients:

- Flour tortillas (as many as required)

Red sauce:

- 4 tbsp. of olive oil
- 1 ½ tsp. of garlic that has been chopped
- 1 ½ cups of readymade tomato puree
- 3 medium tomatoes. Puree them in a mixer
- 1 tsp. of sugar
- A pinch of salt or to the taste
- A few red chili flakes to sprinkle
- 1 tsp. of oregano

Filling:

- 2 tbsp. of oil
- 2 tsp. of chopped garlic
- 2 onions chopped finely
- 2 capsicums chopped finely
- 2 cups of readymade baked beans
- A few drops of Tabasco sauce
- 1 cup of crumbled or roughly mashed cottage cheese (cottage cheese)
- 1 cup of grated cheddar cheese
- A pinch of salt
- 1 tsp. of oregano

- ½ tsp. of pepper
- 1 ½ tsp. of red chili flakes or to taste
- 1 tbsp. of finely chopped jalapenos

To serve:

- 1 cup of grated pizza cheese (mix mozzarella and cheddar cheese)

Directions:

1. Have the tortillas ready to serve.

2. Now, move on to the making of red sauce. Put about 2 teaspoons in a saucepan: apply the garlic to heat and whisk. Under the heading "For the sauce," Keep working, apply the remaining ingredients. Cook until the drops of sauce become dense.

3. To fill another saucepan, heat one tablespoon of oil. Tie the onions and garlic together, then fry until caramelized or golden-brown. Put the remainder of the ingredients into the filling and cook for two minutes.

4. From the flame, take the saucepan and grate some cheese over the pan. Balance well, and allow a little bit of it to settle.

5. Let's get a selection of platters. Take a tortilla, then apply some sauce to the surface. Now place the filling at the right, in a line. Turn the tortilla upwards cautiously. And the same is those around tortillas.

6. Place all the tortillas in a bowl and sprinkle them with the grated cheese. Cover all up with an aluminum board.

7. Preheat at 160 ° C for 4-5 minutes with the Air Fryer. Smash the bowl and the tray inside. At the same time, keep the fryer on for another 15 minutes. Switch the tortillas over in between to get a regular chef.

67.Veg Memo's

Total time: 30 min

Prep time: 10 min

Cook time: 10 min

Yield: 2 servings

Ingredients:

For dough:

- 1 ½ cup of all-purpose flour
- ½ tsp. of salt or to taste
- 5 tbsp. of water

For filling:

- 2 cups of carrots grated
- 2 cups of cabbage grated
- 2 tbsp. of oil
- 2 tsp. of ginger-garlic paste
- 2 tsp. of soy sauce
- 2 tsp. of vinegar

Directions:

1. Setback, knead and cover the dough with plastic wrap. Then, cook the filling ingredients and aim to ensure that the sauce is properly coated with the vegetables.

2. Print the dough out and then slice it into a rectangle. Place the filling in the middle. To safeguard the filling, fold the dough now, then pinch the corners.

3. Preheat at 200 ° F for 5 minutes with the Air Fryer. Place the gnocchi in the frying box and close it. Let them cook at the same time for another 20 minutes. The suggested sides contain chili or sauce with ketchup.

68.Yummy Pollock

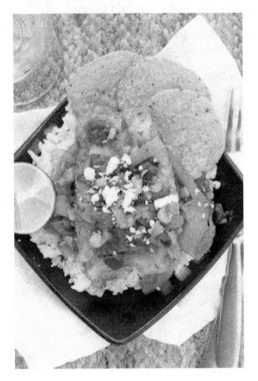

Total time: 25 min

Prep time: 15 min

Cook time: 10 min

Yield: 6 serving

Ingredients:

- Cup 1/2 sour cream
- Four Pollock fillets, barefoot
- Parmesan: 1/4 cup, rubbed
- 2 Mezzanine sugar, melted
- Salt and black chili, to try
- Kitchen spray

Directions:

1. Mix the sour cream in a dish of butter, parmesan, salt and pepper and Whisk well.

2. Sprinkle fish with spray to fry, and season with salt and pepper.

3. Place sour cream mixture on each side. Arrange Pollock fillet in air fryer heated to 350 degrees F, then cook for 15 minutes.

4. Divide Pollock fillets into bowls, and serve with a delightful side salad.

69.Honey Sea Bass

Total time: 40 min

Prep time: 15 min

Cook time: 25 min

Yield: 2 serving

Ingredients:

- 2 Fillets sea bass
- A 1/2 orange zest, rubbed
- 1/2 Fruit juice
- A tablespoon of black pepper and salt
- 2 Mustard spoons
- 2 Honey Teaspoons
- 2 Pounds of olive oil
- 1/2 pound of dried, drained lentils
- A tiny amount of dill, chopped
- 2 Ounces of cress water
- A tiny amount of chopped parsley

Directions:

1. Add salt and peppered fish fillets, apply citrus zest and juice, and rub Rub with 1 spoonful of milk, honey and mustard, and pass to your air Fry and cook for 10 minutes at 350 degrees F, turning in half.

2. In the meantime, place the lentils in a small pot, heat them up over medium heat, and add them Staying with milk, watercress, dill and parsley, mix well and split between

Plates.

3. Insert the fish fillets and serve promptly.

Enjoy it!

Nutrition: 212 calories, 8 fat, 12 fiber, 9 carbohydrates and 17 proteins

70.Tilapia Sauce and Chives
Total time: 20 min

Prep time: 10 min

Cook time: 10 min

Yield: 4 serving

Ingredients:

- 4 Medium fillet with tilapia
- Cooking spray
- Salt and black chili, to satisfy
- 2 Honey Teaspoons
- Greek yoghurt: 1/4 cup
- 1 lemon juice
- 2 Spoonful's of chives, chopped

Directions:

1. Season with salt and pepper, sprinkle with mist, put in

Hot oven 350 degrees F air fryer and cook for ten minutes, tossing

Midway.

2. In the meantime, blend yoghurt with sugar, salt, vinegar, vinegar and chives in a cup

Nice lemon juice and whisk.

3. Divide air fryer fish into bowls, chop yoghurt sauce and serve

Immediately.

Experience!

Nutrition: 261 calories, fat 8, 18 fiber, 24 carbohydrates, 21 protein

71.Tilapia Coconut
Prep time: ten minutes Cooking time: 10 minutes Servings: 4

Ingredients:

- 4 Medium fillet with tilapia
- Salt and black chili, to try
- 1/2 cup of cocoon milk
- 1 Ginger-spoon, rubbed
- Chopped 1/2 cup cilantro
- 2 Sliced cloves of garlic
- 1/2 teaspoon masala garam
- Cooking spray
- Half Jalapeno, Split

Directions:

1. Mix the coconut milk with salt, pepper, cilantro in your food processor, Ginger, garlic, jalapeno which masala garam, and always pulse well.

2. Sprinkle fish with cooking oil, scatter coconut mix around, rub well, Switch to the basket with the air fryer and cook at 400 degrees F for 10 Minutes.

3. Divide between plates, and serve hot.

Experience!

Nutrition: 200 calories, 5 fat, 6 fiber, 25 carbohydrates and 26 protein

72.Catfish fillets special

Total time: 40 min

Prep time: 15 min

Cook time: 25 min

Yield: 5 serving

Ingredients:

- 2 Catfish fillets
- 1/2 Teaspoon of ginger, hazelnut
- 2 Butter on ounces
- Worcestershire 4 ounces sauce

- 1/2 cubicle jerk seasoning
- 1 Mustard casserole
- 1 spoonful of balsamic vinegar
- Catsup: 3/4 cup
- Salt and black chili, to try
- 1 spoonful of parsley, chopped

Directions:

1. Heat up a skillet over medium heat with the butter, add Worcestershire

Seasoning of sauce, garlic, mustard, catsup, vinegar, salt and hot pepper,

Adjust fire, swirl well, and apply fish fillets.

2. Toss well, leave the fillets for 10 minutes, drain them, and pass them to the preheated to 350 degrees F air fryer basket and cook for 8 minutes,

Halfway through flip fillets.

3. Divide into bowls, brush on top with parsley and serve immediately.

73.Tasty French Cod
Total time: 30 min

Prep time: 15 min

Cook time: 15 min

Yield: 6 serving

Ingredients:

- 2 Tsp. of olive oil
- 1 Yellow onion, Sliced
- White wine: 1/2 cup
- 2 cloves of garlic, minced
- 14 Ounces of dried, stewed tomatoes
- Chopped 3 teaspoons of parsley
- 2 Lbs. of cod, boneless
- Salt and black chili, to try
- 2 tablespoons of butter

Directions:

1. Heat a saucepan over medium heat with the oil, add garlic and onion, stir and just cook for five minutes.

2. Add wine, stir and proceed to cook for 1 minute.

3. Stir in tomatoes, bring to a boil, simmer for 2 minutes, add fuel, stir then turn the heat off again.

4. Place this combination into a heat-proof dish that suits your air fryer, add chicken, season with salt and pepper and steam at 350 degrees F in your fryer for 14 minutes.

5. Divide the tomatoes and the fish into plates and serve.

74.Scampi Shrimp and Chips

Preparation Time: 10 Minutes

Cooking Time: 15 Minutes

Servings: 4

Ingredients:

- 2 medium potatoes
- Salt and ground black pepper to taste
- 1 tbsp. olive oil
- 1 lb King prawns
- 1 small egg
- 5 oz. gluten-free oats
- 1 large lemon
- 1 tsp. thyme
- 1 tbsp. parsley

Directions:

1. Cut them into chunky chips after peeling the potatoes, then season with pepper and salt. Drizzle the chip with a little olive oil. Lastly, cook for 5 minutes at 360 F in an air fryer.

2. Rinse the prawns and rinse with a kitchen towel by patting them. To the chopping board, move them and season with pepper and salt.

3. Transfer the egg into a small bowl and blend until you have a beaten egg, using a fork.

4. In the blender, put 80 percent of the gluten-free oats alongside the thyme and parsley. Blend before a paste that looks like coarse breadcrumbs appear to you. Move the mixture to a medium mixing bowl.

5. In another different bowl, add the leftover 20 percent gluten-free oats.

6. Place the prawns in both the blended oats, the egg, and the blended oats.

7. Finally, put the prawns in the oats, which are not blended.

8. Place the chips on the grill pan and extract them from the air fryer.

9. Place the rest of the prawns in the air-fryer grill pan and allow them to cook at 360 F.

10. With fresh lemon juice, season the cooked prawns and chips.

11. Just serve.

75.Gambas 'Pil' with Sweet Potato

Preparation Time: 15 Minutes

Cooking Time: 20 Minutes

Servings: 3-4

Ingredients:

- 12 King prawns
- 4 garlic cloves
- 1 red chili pepper, de-seeded
- 1 shallot
- 4 tbsp. olive oil
- Smoked paprika powder
- 5 large sweet potatoes
- 2 tbsp. olive oil
- 1 tbsp. honey
- 2 tbsp. fresh rosemary, finely chopped
- 4 stalks lemongrass
- 2 limes

Directions:

1. Clean the prawns and gut them.

2. Perfect the garlic and red chili pepper, and chop the shallots.

3. To form a marinade, combine the red chili pepper, garlic, and olive oil alongside the paprika. Let the prawns marinate in the marinade for approximately 2 hours.

4. By cutting the sweet potato, make perfect slices. Using 2 tablespoons of olive oil, honey, and chopped rosemary to mix the potato slices. Inside of an air fryer, bake the potatoes at 360 F for 15 minutes.

5. Thread the prawns onto the lemongrass stalks when baking the potatoes. Increase the temperature to 390 F, and the prawn skewers are also included.

6. Allow 5 minutes to cook the mixture.

7. Serve alongside wedges of lime.

76.Fried Hot Prawns with Cocktail Sauce

Preparation Time: 5 Minutes

Cooking Time: 15 Minutes

Servings: 4

Ingredients:

- 1 tsp. chili powder
- 1 tsp. chili flakes
- ½ tsp. freshly ground black pepper
- ½ tsp. sea salt
- 8-12 fresh king prawns

For sause:

- 1 tbsp. cider or wine vinegar
- 1 tbsp. ketchup
- 3 tbsp. mayonnaise

Directions:

1. Ensure that your Air Fryer is set to 360 F.

2. Get a clean bowl and combine the spices in it.

3. Coat the prawns by tossing them in the spices mixture.

4. Transfer the spicy prawns into the air fryer basket and place the basket in the air fryer.

5. Allow the prawns to cook for 6 to 8 minutes (how long depends on the size of the prawns).

6. Get another clean bowl and make a mixture of the sauce ingredients.

7. Serve the prawns while hot alongside the cocktail sauce.

77. Crispy Air-fryer Coconut Prawns

Preparation Time: 10 Minutes

Cooking Time: 15 Minutes

Servings: 2

Ingredients:

- 1 lb fresh prawns
- 3 oz. granola
- 1 tbsp. Chinese five-spice
- 1 tbsp. mixed spice
- 1 tbsp. coriander
- Salt and ground black pepper to taste
- 1 lime rind and juice
- 2 tbsp. light coconut milk
- 3 tbsp. desiccated coconut
- 1 small egg

Directions:

1. After cleaning your prawns, lay them out on a chopping board.

2. Blend the granola in a blender until it appears like fine breadcrumbs.

3. Before removing the granola blend from the blender, add all the seasonings, lime, and coconut mix.

4. Whizz the blender around again.

5. Get a clean bowl and beat your egg in it using a fork.

6. While holding each prawn by the tail, dip it into the egg and the batter one after another.

7. After dipping all the prawns line the baking sheet at the bottom of the air fryer with your prawns.

8. Allow cooking at 360 F for 18 minutes.

9. Serve the cooked prawns.

11. King Prawns in Ham with Red Pepper Dip

Preparation Time: 10 Minutes

Cooking Time: 20 Minutes

Servings: 10

Ingredients:

- 1 large red bell pepper, halved
- 10 (frozen) king prawns, defrosted
- 5 slices of raw ham
- 1 tbsp. olive oil
- ½ tbsp. paprika
- 1 large clove garlic, crushed
- Salt to taste
- Freshly ground black pepper to taste
- Tapas forks

Directions:

1. Ensure the heating process of the air fryer to 390 F.

2. Place the bell pepper in the basket of the air fryer and let it roast for 10 minutes; extract when the skin is finely charred.

3. In a bowl, move the roasted bell pepper when covering it with an adhesive film or lid. Allow it for about 15 minutes to relax.

4. To allow you to take the black vein out, peel your prawns and make a deep incision in the back. Lengthwise, cut the ham into strips, and wrap each prawn in each slice of ham.

5. Using a thin film of olive oil to cover each parcel and transfer it into the basket. Place the basket back in the air fryer and let fry for 3 minutes. Once the prawns appear crispy and just right, withdraw.

6. Peel off the skin of the bell pepper halves while frying the prawns, and get rid of the seeds too. Then cut the pepper into bits and, besides olive oil, paprika, and garlic, purée the pieces in the blender. In a dish, pass the sauce and add pepper and salt to taste.

7. Serve in a pan alongside tapas forks the prawns in damage. A little dish of red pepper dip should be included.

78. Crispy Crabstick Crackers

Preparation Time: 10 Minutes

Cooking Time: 15 Minutes

Servings: 2-3

Ingredients:

- 1 packet Crabstick Filament, thawed
- Cooking Spray

Directions:

1. Ensure that the setting of your Air Fryer is 360 F.

2. Peel and unrolled them after detaching the plastic wrapping on of crabstick filament. Finally, separate them into small pieces, which is good for thicker crackers 1/2 inch wide.

3. Spray them with a cooking spray before moving them into the frying basket.

4. Transfer the crab sticks to the air fryer in batches.

5. For 8-10 minutes, air fry each batch.

6. Remove the tray in the fourth minute and stir the crabstick crackers with the kitchen tongs, which ensures they do not stick together.

7. Adjust and allow to cool before storing them in an airtight container when air frying is completed.

79.Wasabi Crab Cakes

Preparation Time: 10 Minutes

Cooking Time: 25 Minutes

Servings: 2

Ingredients:

- 2 large egg whites

- 1 celery rib, finely chopped
- 1 medium sweet red pepper, finely chopped
- 3 green onions, finely chopped
- ¼ tsp. prepared wasabi
- 3 tbsp. reduced-fat mayonnaise
- ¼ tsp. salt
- 1/3 cup plus ½ cup dry bread crumbs, divided
- 1-1/2 cups lump crabmeat, drained
- Cooking spray

Sauce:

- ½ tsp. prepared wasabi
- 1 green onion, chopped
- 1 celery rib, chopped
- 1 tbsp. sweet pickle relish
- ¼ tsp. celery salt
- 1/3 cup reduced-fat mayonnaise

Directions:

1. Make sure the Air Fryer is preheated to 375 F and that the basket of the air fryer is sprayed with cooking spray.

2. Get a bowl and, along with 1/3 cup breadcrumbs, make a mixture of the first seven ingredients. Fold in the crab softly.

3. Take a shallow bowl and place in the remaining bread crumbs. Then add the bowl of heaping tablespoonful of crab mixture. Coat and shape the crumbs into 3/4-inch-thick patties.

4. If required, you should operate in samples batch of crab cakes should be arranged to form a single layer in the air fryer basket.

5. Just cook with cooking spray after spritzing the crab cakes.

6. It should take about 8 to 12 minutes to cook, or until the cakes turn golden brown. Turn the cakes halfway through heating, then spritz again with extra cooking oil.

7. Withdraw and keep warm once cooked.

8. For the other batches, do the same.

9. Place the sauce ingredients in your food processor while cooking the cakes, and blend to the preferred consistency.

10. In addition to the dipping sauce, serve fried crabs while warm.

80.Flourless Truly Crispy Calamari Rings

Preparation Time: 05 Minutes

Cooking Time: 10 Minutes

Servings: 2

Ingredients:

- 1 oz. calamari
- 1 cup gluten-free oats
- 1 large egg, beaten
- 1 tbsp. paprika
- 1 tsp. parsley
- 1 small lemon juice and rind
- Salt and ground black pepper to taste

Directions:

1. Ensure that your Air Fryer is preheated to 360 F.

2. Slice your calamari thinly to produce small rings of calamari.

3. Using a food processor or a blender, blend your oats until you have a consistency that looks like that of fine breadcrumbs.

4. Transfer the beaten egg to a separate bowl and the oats to another bowl.

5. Mix the oats with paprika and parsley.

6. Get a chopping board, and coat your calamari rings on it using salt, lemon, and pepper.

7. Your hands may be sticky; thus, ensure you rub them in the oats.

8. Transfer the calamari rings into the oats first, then into the egg, then the oats, why ensuring that they are thoroughly coated at each stage.

9. Get rid of any excess oats and transfer the rings into the baking mat of your air fryer.

10. Allow cooking for 8 minutes at 360 F.

11. Serve!

81.Scallops Wrapped in Bacon

Preparation Time: 10 Minutes

Cooking Time: 15 Minutes

Servings: 4

Ingredients:

- 8 scallops
- 8 bacon slices
- Toothpicks

Directions:

1. Wrap the bacon over the scallop.

2. Hold it in place with a toothpick.

3. Set your air fryer to 360 F and air fry the bacon.

4. Withdraw after 18 minutes or when a beautiful golden brown color is observed.

82.Tilapia Fillet with Vegetables
Preparation Time: 20 Minutes

Cooking Time: 40 Minutes

Servings: 2

Ingredients:

- 2 tilapia fillets Mushrooms to taste
- 1 broccoli
- 1 sweet potato
- 1 carrot Seasoning to taste

Directions:

1. Grill and sauté the mushrooms in the oil.

2. Cut the vegetables, season and place on a baking sheet and close with laminated paper.

3. Baked it in the fryer at 4000F for 25 minutes.

4. Make a beautiful dish and have a good appetite.

83.Shrimps in the Pumpkin

Preparation Time: 10 Minutes

Cooking Time: 30 Minutes

Servings: 4

Ingredients:

- 2 ¼ lb of medium shrimp
- 4 tbsp. of olive oil
- 2 cloves of garlic
- 1 onion
- 5 seedless tomatoes, Salt and black pepper to taste.
- 1 can of cream without serum
- ½ lb of cream cheese
- 1 strawberry
- green aroma to taste
- 3 tbsp. of tomato sauce

Directions:

1. Remove the top and the strawberry seeds.

2. Wash and seal in foil and bake at 360 ° F for 45 minutes in an air fryer.

3. Heat the oil and sauté the garlic and onion in a saucepan, add the shrimp, and cook for 5 minutes.

4. Stir in the diced tomatoes, salt, pepper and tomato sauce.

5. Turn the heat off and apply the green smell and cream.

6. Mix well, and then apply the curd.

7. Place the strawberry inside a bit of curd and pour the shrimp cream.

84.Shrimp Strogonoff
Preparation Time: 10 Minutes

Cooking Time: 15 Minutes

Servings: 2-4

Ingredients:

- 1 tbsp. butter 1 medium
- Onion grated

- 1 lb of medium clean shrimp

- Salt and pepper

- 4 tbsp. of brandy

- 3 ½ oz. minced pickled mushrooms

- 3 tbsp. of tomato sauce

- 1 tbsp. of mustard

- 1 can of cream set aside.

Directions:

1. Make the shrimp clean. Remove the peels and use water and lemon to wash them very well.

2. Heat the onion butter and brown it. Season with salt and pepper, remove from the heat and blend with the shrimp and stir well.

3. Put the fryer in the air for 5 minutes at 3200F.

4. In a shell, heat the cognac until it catches fire. Then spill it over the burning shrimp.

5. Add the mushroom, tomato sauce, mustard and cook for about 5 minutes in an air fryer.

6. Add the milk before serving, stir well and steam without boiling. 7. Use white rice and straw potatoes to eat the stroganoff.

85.Pumpkin Shrimp with Catupiry
Preparation Time: 20 Minutes

Cooking Time: 30 Minutes

Servings: 2-4

Ingredients:

- 1 large strawberry

- 2 ¼ lb of medium shrimp

- 1 pot of catupiry

- 1 glass of palm heart

- 1 bottle of coconut milk Salt Chile

- 1 grated onion

- 2 cloves of garlic

- 2 chopped seedless tomatoes
- 1 tbsp. of wheat flour dessert

Directions:

1. Remove the cap of the strawberry and all the seeds then. Spray salt on the interior after cleaning. Wrap the aluminum foil around the whole strawberry. Bake at 4000F in an air-fryer for 45 minutes. Set back, but before using a spoon, add some strawberry slices to the stew.

2. In the fat, cook the onion and garlic. Then she took out the tomatoes and strawberry slices, leaving them too steep for 10 minutes. Attach the sliced palm kernel and then the shrimp that you shouldn't cook for more than 10 minutes, so it's going to be completely hard if you cook it longer. To make it slightly thick, add the coconut milk and 1 tablespoon of flour dissolved in water. And apply half the catupiry box to the prepared stir fry and turn off, mixing it well into the stir fry and salt.

3. Take catupiry balls with your hands with the strawberry still hot and put them on the bottom and sides (the catupiry must be very cold to stick more easily).

4. Pour in the strawberry with the hot stir fry and eat.

5. Put in parsley or coriander to taste (it depends on the flavor of each one).

86.Fricassee of Jamila Shrimps
Preparation Time: 15 Minutes

Cooking Time: 40 Minutes

Servings: 2-5

Ingredients:

- 2 ¼ lb clean shrimp
- Salt and pepper to taste olive oil
- 1 large grated onion Chopped garlic
- 3 tomatoes, chopped parsley and chives
- 1 can of vegetable
- 1 can of sour cream
- 1 can of corn grated
- cheese to taste
- 2 glasses of curd

- ½ lb mozzarella cheese
- potato sticks

Directions:

1. Wash the shrimp and season with salt, pepper and lemon. Allow time for the seasoning to soak in.

2. Sauté the grated onion, minced garlic, tomatoes, parsley, and chives in olive oil.

3. Add the shrimp and the garden. Mix and cook for about 5 minutes or until shrimp are pink. Reserve.

4. Whisk the corn with sour cream and grated cheese in a blender.

5. Spread the creamy curd, shrimp sauce on a plate, and then pour the whipped cream on top.

6. Cover with mozzarella.

7. Take to the air fryer to brown at 3600F for 30 minutes.

8. Serve hot with white rice and straw potatoes.

87.Fried Beach Shrimps
Preparation Time: 5 Minutes

Cooking Time: 15 Minutes

Servings: 2-4

Ingredients:

- 2 ¼ lb of clean and washed gray shrimp
- ½ lemon Salt 1
- ½ tbsp. of flour
- 2 garlic cloves, squeezed

Directions:

1. Season shrimp (must be very dry) with salt, lemon, and squeezed garlic.

2. Sprinkle the flour and mix well.

3. Take to the air fryer at 3600F for 15 minutes and fry until golden. Serve well with a leafy salad and white rice.

88.Fried Shrimp without Flour

Preparation Time: 5 Minutes

Cooking Time: 10 Minutes

Servings: 2

Ingredients:

- ½ lb small shrimp without shell
- 2 tbsp. of olive oil
- 2 garlic cloves, crushed
- ½ large onion, chopped
- 2 tbsp. soy sauce salt to taste black pepper to taste

Directions:

1. In a pan, add a little olive oil, crushed garlic, and onion, marinate for 5 minutes.

2. Add the shrimp, salt, black pepper, and soy sauce.

3. Take to the air fryer at 3600 F. Let it cook for 10 minutes.

4. Let shrimp fry until golden brown, then sprinkle with Parmesan cheese.

5. Parsley to taste grated fresh parmesan cheese to taste

89.Shrimps with Garlic and Oil
Preparation Time: 10 Minutes

Cooking Time: 15 Minutes

Servings: 4-6

Ingredients:

- 3 lbs. medium shrimp
- 10 cloves of garlic
- Salt to taste
- Olive oil to taste

Directions:

1. Wash the shrimp in the shell, with the head removed.

2. Peel the cloves of garlic, and cut them in half.

3. Fry the garlic in the oil well (well done).

4. Place the shrimp in a saucepan and sprinkle it with some salt.

5. Take it to the 3200F air fryer for 5 minutes.

6. Place the oil in a bowl with the garlic and pour it over it.

7. Serve with beer with snow.

90.Breaded Prawns
Preparation Time: 5 Minutes

Cooking Time: 15 Minutes

Servings: 1-2

Ingredients:

- 12 large prawns
- 3 tablespoons butter, melted
- 6 eggs Wheat flour to the point Salt to taste
- 1 tbsp. of virgin olive oil

Directions:

1. Cook the prawns in the air fryer at 3200F, being careful not to cook them for about 10 minutes. Remove.

2. Then peel the prawns and place them in the melted butter, resting.

3. Separate the whites from the yolks of the 6 eggs, beating the whites in the snow, then add the wheat flour until it sighs, season with salt and the spoon of oil.

4. Then, place the prawns in this pasta and with a spoon, remove each shrimp, accompanied by a little pasta.

5. Put back in the air fryer for 5 minutes.

91. Vegetable Supreme Pan Pizza

Preparation Time: 15 Minutes

Cooking Time: 30 Minutes

Servings: 3

Ingredients:

- 8 slice White Onion
- 12 slice Tomato
- 2 tablespoon olive oil
- 3/2 cup shredded mozzarella
- 8 Cremini mushrooms
- 1/2 green pepper
- 4 tablespoon Pesto
- 1 Pizza Dough
- 1 cup spinach

Directions:

1. Roll the pizza dough halves until they each meet the size of the Air Flow racks.

2. Grease all sides of each dough lightly with olive oil.

3. On a rack, put each pizza. Place the racks on the electric fryer's upper and lower shelves.

4. Then press the power button and the cooking time to 13 minutes by pressing the French Fries button (400° F).

5. Flip the dough onto the top shelf after 5 minutes and switch the racks.

6. Switch the dough on to the top shelf after 4 minutes.

7. Take both racks out and drizzle the toppings with the pizzas.

8. Place the racks on the electric fryer's upper and lower shelves.

9. Then push the power button and the cooking time to 7 minutes by pressing the French Fries button (400° F).

10. Rotate the pizzas after 4 minutes.

11. If the pizzas are done, let them rest before cutting them for 4 minutes.

92. Pignoli Cookies

Preparation Time: 15 Minutes

Cooking Time: 25 Minutes

Servings: 36

Ingredients:

- 2 cup pine nuts

- 4 large egg whites
- 1 cup confectioners' sugar
- 1/2 cup sugar
- 10-ounce almond paste

Directions:

1. In a bowl, whisk the almond paste and sugar together until just mixed.

2. Through the almond mixture, add 2 egg whites.

3. Add the confectioner's sugar to the almond mixture gradually and blend well to form a dough.

4. Until the whites are foamy, pound the remaining two egg whites in a separate bowl.

5. To prevent the dough from sticking to your fingers, dip your fingers in the flour. Shape 1 inch into the dough. In the egg whites, dip the balls and coat each ball with the pine nuts.

6. Place the balls and flatten each ball gently on two parchment-lined Air Flow Racks.

7. On the bottom and middle shelves of the appliance, place the racks.

8. Press the power button, the cooking temperature is lowered to 325 ° F, and the cooking time is increased to 18 minutes. Switch racks in the middle of cooking time (9 minutes).

93. Jam Filled Buttermilk Scones

Preparation Time: 15 Minutes

Cooking Time: 25 Minutes

Servings: 6

Ingredients:

- 2¼ cup flour
- 1 teaspoon salt
- 1/4 cup sugar
- 2 teaspoon Baking Powder
- 12 tablespoon butter
- 2 large eggs
- 1/3 cup buttermilk

- 1 teaspoon Vanilla Extract
- 1/2 cup strawberry jams
- 2 tablespoon demerara sugar

Directions:

1. In a container, mix the baking powder, flour, sugar and salt together.

2. Using the wider holes on a box grater, grind the butter into the dish.

3. Combine the cup with the ingredients.

4. To complete the dough, whisk together the patted eggs, vanilla, and buttermilk into the bowl.

5. Break the dough in two, form each half of the dough into a disc, cover the discs with plastic wrap and put them in the fridge for 60 minutes.

6. Using a fresh sheet of plastic wrap to position a disc. Roll the disc to a thickness of 1/2 inch.

7. Spread the jam on the disk leaving a ½ in. scab around the edges.

8. Roll the other disc to 1/2-inch thickness into another layer of plastic wrap.

9. Place the second discover the first disc and press softly to secure the discs' edges.

10. Made into eight wedges with the dough.

11. On two parchment-lined Air Flow shelves, put shims. Brush the wedges with the buttermilk generously and dust with the Demerara sugar. Place the racks on the appliance's bottom and center shelves.

12. Press the power button to raise the cooking temperature to 375 degrees F and simmer for 18 minutes. After 10 mins, rotate the shelves.

94. Chicken Milanese

Preparation Time: 10 Minutes

Cooking Time: 20 Minutes

Servings: 3

Ingredients:

- 4 chicken cutlets
- 2 tablespoon Extra Virgin Olive Oil
- Juice of 1/2 lemon
- Shaved parmesan for garnish

- 2 cup panko breadcrumbs
- 2 eggs, beaten
- 1 teaspoon Garlic powder
- 1 beefsteak tomato, diced
- Salt and black pepper, divided
- 3 cup arugula
- 1/4 cup parmesan, grated
- 1 teaspoon White wine vinegar

Directions:

1. Bring the panko breadcrumbs, parmesan, and garlic powder together in a dish.

2. With salt and pepper, softly season the chicken cutlets.

3. In a separate bowl, add the eggs.

4. Through the egg, drop the cutlets. Then coat the panko mixture with it.

5. On the Air Flow Racks, position the cutlets

6. Click the Button for Steaks/Chops (370°F). To start the cooking cycle, reduce the cooking time to 15 minutes.

7. Prepare the salad when the chicken is preparing food: stir in the lemon juice, olive oil, vinegar and a pinch of salt and pepper in a container.

8. Use the dressing to add the arugula and coat.

9. Place the chicken on a plate when the chicken is done eating and top with the chopped tomato and the arugula salad, and top with the shaved Parmesan.

95. White Pizza
Preparation Time: 15 Minutes

Cooking Time: 25 Minutes

Servings: 1

Ingredients:

- 2 clove garlic, thinly sliced
- 1 thin-crust pizza dough
- 9 slice fresh mozzarella

- 1 teaspoon red pepper flakes

- 1/4 cup ricotta cheese

- 2 tablespoon extra-virgin olive oil, divided

Directions:

1. Use 1 tablespoon of olive oil to rub the pizza dough. To suit on an Air Flow rack, roll the pizza dough out.

2. Put the pizza on the rack and slide it onto the Air Fryer oven center shelf.

3. Press the control button and then the (400 ° F / 200 ° C) French Fries button. To begin the cooking cycle, you manually set the cooking time to 10 minutes. Turn the dough over halfway through the cooking time (5 minutes).

4. From the Air Fryer oven, remove the crust.

5. Drizzle the ricotta, mozzarella, garlic and red pepper flakes with the crust. Bring the pizza back to the Power Air Fryer oven.

6. Press the control button and then the (400 ° F / 200 ° C) French Fries button. To begin the cooking cycle, you manually set the cooking time to 6 minutes. Cook until you've melted the cheese.

7. One teaspoon Drizzle. Before eating, place olive oil on the pizza.

96. Cheddar Biscuits
Preparation Time: 10 Minutes

Cooking Time: 30 Minutes

Servings: 16

Ingredients:

- 3/4 cup buttermilk

- 1/2 teaspoon seafood seasoning

- 1/2 cup scallions, chopped

- 1/4 teaspoon Cayenne powder

- 2 cup flour

- 1 stick butter

- 2 teaspoon Baking Powder
- 3/2 cup cheddar, shredded

Directions:

1. In a bowl, combine the flour and butter until it is pea-size.

2. Add the remaining ingredients and whisk.

3. Divide into 16 balls and place in an Air Flow Rack.

4. Press the baking button. Reduce the timer to 15 minutes to start the cook cycle.

5. Serve.

97. Maryland Crab Cakes
Preparation Time: 10 Minutes

Cooking Time: 20 Minutes

Servings: 5

Ingredients:

- 1 teaspoon salt
- 1 cup cracker crumbs
- 1 pound Lump crab meat
- 1 pinch salt and pepper to season
- 2 tablespoon fresh parsley, chopped
- 1 teaspoon seafood seasoning
- 1/2 teaspoon ground black pepper
- 1/4 cup scallions, finely chopped
- 1 tablespoon sweet chili sauce
- 1 teaspoon garlic, minced
- 1 cup mayonnaise
- 1 tablespoon sweet pickle relish
- 1/4 cup Celery, diced
- 1 tablespoon Lemon juice
- 1 tablespoon Thai chili sauce

Directions:

1. In a large bowl, bring together all the breadcrumb ingredients except the crabmeat and cookie crumbs.

2. Gently mix the crab meat and 1/4 cup of the cracker crumbs.

3. Spread the remaining crumbs out on a work surface.

4. Form 12 equal-sized balls with crab mixture.

5. Place the balls on top of the crumbs to coat evenly and press gently to make a patty.

6. Place in a refrigerator for 20 minutes.

7. Place the crab cakes on the Air Flow racks.

8. Press the Steaks / Chops button. Reduce the timer to 20 minutes to begin the cook cycle.

9. While the crab cakes are cooking, prepare the dipping sauce: combine all the ingredients and season with salt and pepper.

10. Serve hot crab cakes with dipping sauce.

98. Pepperoni Stuffed Mozzarella Patties

Preparation Time: 15 Minutes

Cooking Time: 30 Minutes

Servings: 12

Ingredients:

- 2 cup seasoned Italian breadcrumbs
- 24 slice pepperonis
- 1-pound whole milk mozzarella
- 4 eggs beaten

Directions:

1. Cut a mozzarella block into 1/4-inch slices. Chop each slice in half.

2. Place two pepperoni slices over the middle of the slices.

3. Create a cheese sandwich with the rest of the mozzarella halves and press tightly to seal.

4. Prepare a dredging station using flour, eggs and breadcrumbs. Dip each mozzarella sandwich in the flour, then the egg, then the breadcrumbs. Once more, dip each sandwich back into the egg and then into the breadcrumbs.

5. Sprinkle patties with cooking spray.

6. Cook sandwiches in the Air Fryer Oven at 400 degrees F for 6 minutes, turning patties midway through cooking.

99. Corned Beef and Cabbage Egg Rolls
Preparation Time: 10 Minutes

Cooking Time: 20 Minutes

Servings: 12

Ingredients:

- 3/2 cup stewed cabbage
- 12 egg roll wrappers
- 3/4-pound corned beef, shredded
- Spicy Mustard

Directions:

1. Working with one egg roll wrapper at a time, position the wrap with one corner of the wrap facing you.

2. Use about 2 tablespoons of minced corned beef to create a small log in the middle of the wrapper. Top the corned beef with 1 tablespoon shredded cabbage. Roll the corner of the egg roll wrapper over the filling and cautiously fold in the wrapper to form an airtight seal.

3. Scrub the rest of the edges of the wrapper with water. Fold each side of the wrap and then roll the egg roll to seal. Redo until all the meat and cabbage are gone.

4. Position the egg rolls on an Air Flow rack. Spray muffins with cooking spray. Slide the rack onto the center shelf of the Air Fryer oven. Press the French fry's button (400°F), set the cooking time to 7 minutes and cook until golden brown.

5. When the egg rolls are done, serve them warm with spicy mustard.

100. Fish Tacos
Preparation Time: 10 Minutes

Cooking Time: 30 Minutes

Servings: 6

Ingredients:

- 6 flour tortillas
- 1 cup coleslaw
- 1 cup panko breadcrumbs
- 1/2 cup salsa
- 1/2 cup guacamole
- 1 cup flour
- 3/2 cup seltzer water, cold
- 2 tablespoon cilantros, chopped
- 1 lemon, cut into wedges
- 10-ounce cod filet
- 1 teaspoon ground white pepper
- 1 tablespoon Cornstarch
- Salt, to taste, divided

Directions:

Tempura Batter:

1. In a bowl, bring together the flour, cornstarch and salt.

2. Mix in the cold seltzer.

3. Mix all the ingredients until consistency is attained.

Taco:

1. Cut the cod fillet into long 2-oz. pieces and season with salt and white pepper.

2. In a skillet: Add the panko breadcrumbs. Dip each piece of cod in the tempura batter. Next, dredge the cod in the panko breadcrumbs.

3. Position the breaded cod on the Air Flow racks. Slide racks into Power Air Fryer oven.

4. Set the appliance to the French fries setting (400°F). Set the cooking time to 10 minutes.

5. Midway through the cook cycle, turn the fish sticks.

6. Once the cooking time is over, remove the fish rods.

7. Spread the guacamole on a tortilla. Place a fish stick on the tortilla and top with some coleslaw, salsa, and a dash of lemon. Top with chopped cilantro.

8. Repeat until all ingredients are used up.

9. Fold the tacos before eating.

Conclusion

You already know that if you have an air fryer, it's a futuristic gadget designed to save time and make you live easier. You'll be excited to hear about how soon you'll be addicted to use your air fryer to cook almost every meal if you've still not taken the jump. Don't think much and kick start a healthy living. This book will provide you with lots of amazing recipes to make using your air fryer.

The Air Fryer Recipes

How to Prepare Easy and Healthy Recipes for Quick And Easy Meals

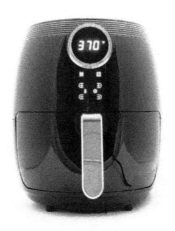

Introduction

In the frying process, the Air Fryer is nothing but a groundbreaking invention and is a user-friendly device. It is essentially a frying machine that can use hot air to fry, bake or roast food and does not require any oil, although it also does not apply any oil to food. This ensures that the food that you fry stays free of calories and oil.

The Air Fryer lets you cook, roast, barbecue, and steam healthier, easier, and more effectively. As many others around the world do, we hope you enjoy using the Air Fryer, and the recipes inside inspire you to cook healthy, well-balanced meals for you and your family.

Air Fryer Recipes

1.Mini Veggie Quiche Cups

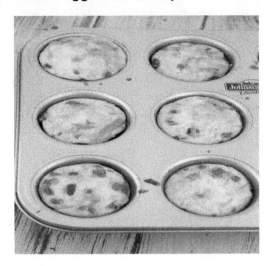

Total time: 30 min

Prep time: 10 min

Cook time: 20 min

Yield: 12 servings

Ingredients:

- 8 eggs
- 3/4 cup cheddar cheese, shredded
- 10 oz. frozen spinach, chopped
- 1/4 cup onion, chopped
- 1/4 cup mushroom, diced
- 1/4 cup bell pepper, diced

Directions:

4. Spray 12 cups muffin pan with cooking spray and set aside.

5. Insert wire rack in rack position 6. Select bake, set temperature 375 f, timer for 20 minutes. Press start to preheat the oven.

6. Add all ingredients into the mixing bowl and beat until combine.

117

7. Pour egg mixture into the prepared muffin pan and bake for 20 minutes.

8. Serve and enjoy.

9.

2.Lemon Blueberry Muffins

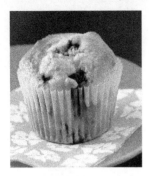

Total time: 35 min

Prep time: 10 min

Cook time: 25 min

Yield: 12 servings

Ingredients:

- 2 eggs
- 1 tsp. baking powder
- 5 drops stevia
- 1/4 cup butter, melted
- 1 cup heavy whipping cream
- 2 cups almond flour
- 1/4 tsp. lemon zest
- 1/2 tsp. lemon extract
- 1/2 cup fresh blueberries

Directions:

1. Spray the muffin pan with 12 cups of cooking spray and set it aside.
2. Wire rack insertion at rack position 6. Pick bake, set temperature to 350 f, 25-minute timer. To preheat the oven, press start.

3. Whisk the eggs together in a mixing dish.

4. Apply the remaining ingredients to the eggs and combine until well mixed.

5. In the prepared muffin tin, add flour and bake for 25 minutes.

6. Enjoy and serve.

3.Baked Breakfast Donuts

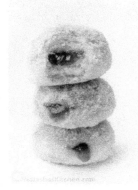

Total time: 30 min

Prep time: 10 min

Cook time: 20 min

Yield: 6 servings

Ingredients:

- 4 eggs
- 1/3 cup almond milk
- 1 tbsp. liquid stevia
- 3 tbsp. cocoa powder
- 1/4 cup coconut oil
- 1/3 cup coconut flour
- 1/2 tsp. baking soda
- 1/2 tsp. baking powder
- 1/2 tsp. instant coffee

Directions:

1. Spray donut pan with cooking spray and set aside.

2. Insert wire rack in rack position 6. Select bake, set temperature 350 f, timer for 20 minutes. Press start to preheat the oven.

3. Add all ingredients into the mixing bowl and mix until well combined.

4. Pour batter into the donut pan and bake for 20 minutes.

5. Serve and enjoy.

4.Blueberry Almond Muffins

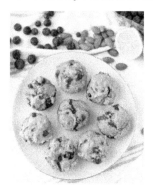

Total time: 25 min

Prep time: 10 min

Cook time: 15 min

Yield: 8 servings

Ingredients:

- 1 egg
- 5 drops liquid stevia
- 1/4 tsp. vanilla extract
- 3/4 cup heavy cream
- 1/4 cup butter
- 1/2 cup fresh blueberries
- 1/2 tsp. baking soda
- 1/4 tsp. baking powder

- 2 1/2 cup almond flour
- 1/2 tsp. salt

Directions:

10. Spray 8 cups muffin pan with cooking spray and set aside.
11. Insert wire rack in rack position 6. Select bake, set temperature 375 f, timer for 15 minutes. Press start to preheat the oven.
12. In a bowl, mix together almond flour, salt, and baking powder.
13. In a large bowl, whisk together egg, butter, vanilla, stevia, baking soda, and heavy cream.
14. Add almond flour mixture into the egg mixture and stir to combine.
15. Pour batter into the muffin pan and bake for 15 minutes.
16. Serve and enjoy.

5.Feta Broccoli Frittata

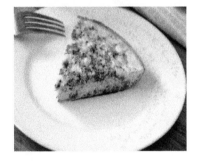

Total time: 30 min

Prep time: 10 min

Cook time: 20 min

Yield: 4 servings

Ingredients:

- 10 eggs
- 2 oz. feta cheese, crumbled
- 2 cups broccoli florets, chopped

- 1 tomato, diced
- 1 tsp. black pepper
- 1 tsp. salt

Directions:

1. Grease baking dish with butter and set aside.

2. Insert wire rack in rack position 6. Select bake, set temperature 390 f, timer for 20 minutes. Press start to preheat the oven.

3. In a bowl, whisk eggs, pepper, and salt. Add veggies and stir well.

4. Pour egg mixture into the baking dish and sprinkle with crumbled cheese.

5. Bake for 20 minutes.

6. Serve and enjoy.

6.Creamy Spinach Quiche

Total time: 45 min

Prep time: 10 min

Cook time: 35 min

Yield: 6 servings

Ingredients:

- 10 eggs
- 1 cup heavy cream
- 1 tbsp. butter
- 1/4 cup fresh scallions, minced
- 1 cup cheddar cheese, shredded
- 1/4 tsp. pepper
- 1/4 tsp. salt
- 1 cup fresh spinach
- 1 cup of coconut milk

Directions:

1. Spray 9*13-inch baking pan with cooking spray and set aside.
2. Insert wire rack in rack position 6. Select bake, set temperature 350 f, timer for 35 minutes. Press start to preheat the oven.
3. In a bowl, whisk eggs, cream, coconut milk, pepper, and salt.
4. Pour egg mixture into the baking pan and sprinkle with spinach, scallions, and cheese.
5. Bake for 35 minutes.
6. Serve and enjoy.

7.Turkey and Quinoa Stuffed Peppers

Total time: 50 min

Prep time: 15 min

Cook time: 35 min

Yield: 6 servings

Ingredients:

- 3 large red bell peppers
- 2 tsp. Chopped fresh rosemary
- 2 tbsp. Chopped fresh parsley
- 3 tbsp. Chopped pecans, toasted
- 2 tbsp. Extra virgin olive oil
- ½ cup chicken stock
- ½ lb. Fully cooked smoked turkey sausage, diced
- ½ tsp. Salt
- 2 cups water
- 1 cup uncooked quinoa

Directions:

1. Place a large saucepan on a high flame and add salt, water and quinoa. Just get it to a boil.

2. Reduce the fire to a simmer after boiling, cover and cook until all the water is consumed for about 15 minutes.

3. Switch off the fire and let it stand for another 5 minutes. Uncover the quinoa.

4. Lengthwise, break the peppers in half and remove the membranes and seeds. Add the peppers to another boiling pot of water, cook for 5 minutes, rinse and discard the water.

5. Grease a 13 x 9 baking dish and preheat the oven to 350.

6. Put the boiling bell pepper on the prepared baking dish, fill the quinoa mixture evenly and pop it into the oven.

7. For 15 minutes, roast.

8.Curried Chicken, Chickpeas and Raito Salad

Prep time: 10 minutes

Cook time: 30 minutes

Yield: 5 servings

Ingredients:

- 1 cup red grapes, halved
- 3-4 cups rotisserie chicken, meat coarsely shredded
- 2 tbsp. Cilantro
- 1 cup plain yogurt
- 2 medium tomatoes, chopped
- 1 tsp. ground cumin
- 1 tbsp. Curry powder
- 2 tbsp. Vegetable oil
- 1 tbsp. Minced peeled ginger
- 1 tbsp. Minced garlic
- 1 medium onion, chopped
- Chickpeas ingredients:
- ¼ tsp. Cayenne
- ½ tsp. Turmeric
- 1 tsp. ground cumin
- 1 19-oz can chickpeas, rinsed, drained and patted dry
- 1 tbsp. Vegetable oil
- Topping and ratio ingredients:
- ½ cup sliced and toasted almonds
- 2 tbsp. Chopped mint
- 2 cups cucumber, peeled, cored and chopped
- 1 cup plain yogurt

Directions:

1. To make the chicken salad, on medium-low fire, place a medium nonstick saucepan and heat oil.

2. Sauté ginger, garlic and onion for 5 minutes or until softened while stirring occasionally.

3. Add 1 ½ tsp. Salt, cumin and curry. Sauté for two minutes.

4. Increase fire to medium-high and add tomatoes. Stirring frequently, cook for 5 minutes.

5. Pour sauce into a bowl, mix in chicken, cilantro and yogurt. Stir to combine and let it stand to cool to room temperature.

6. To make the chickpeas, on a nonstick fry pan, heat oil for 3 minutes.

7. Add chickpeas and cook for a minute while stirring almost continually.

8. Add ¼ tsp. Salt, cayenne, turmeric and cumin. Stir to mix well and cook for two minutes or until sauce is dried.

9. Transfer to a bowl and let it cool to room temperature.

10. To make the ratio, mix ½ tsp. salt, mint, cucumber and yogurt. Stir thoroughly to combine and dissolve the salt.

11. To assemble, in four 16-oz lidded jars or bowls, layer the following: curried chicken, ratio, chickpeas, and garnish with almonds.

12. You can make this recipe one day ahead and refrigerate for 6 hours before serving.

9.Balsamic Vinaigrette on Roasted Chicken

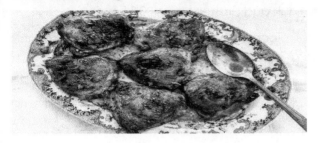

Total time: 1 hour 10 min

Prep time: 10 min

Cook time: 60 min

Yield: 8 servings

Ingredients:

- 1 tbsp. Chopped fresh parsley
- 1 tsp. Lemon zest
- ½ cup low-salt chicken broth
- One 4-lb whole chicken, cut into pieces
- Freshly ground black pepper
- Salt
- 2 tbsp. Olive oil
- 2 garlic cloves, chopped
- 2 tbsp. Fresh lemon juice
- 2 tbsp. Dijon mustard
- ¼ cup balsamic vinegar

Directions:

1. Whisk together the pepper, salt, olive oil, garlic, lemon juice, mustard and vinegar in a small cup.

2. Combine the above mixture and the chicken parts in a re-sealable bag. Refrigerate for at least 2 hours or a whole day and

marinate. Make sure that the bag is turned upside-down sometimes.

3. Grease a baking dish and preheat the 400 ° f oven.

4. Place marinated pieces of chicken on a baking dish and popped them into the oven.

5. Roast the chicken for an hour or until fully baked. Cover with foil if the chicken is browned and not yet completely baked, and finish cooking.

6. Take the chicken out of the oven and pass it to a serving dish.

7. Garnish with parsley and, before eating, drizzle with lemon juice.

10. Chicken Pasta Parmesan

Total time: 30 min

Prep time: 10 min

Cook time: 20 min

Yield: 1 servings

Ingredients:

- ½ cup cooked whole-wheat spaghetti

- 1 oz. Reduced-fat mozzarella cheese, grated

- ¼ cup prepared marinara sauce

- 2 tbsp. Seasoned dry breadcrumbs

- 4 oz. Skinless chicken breast

- 1 tbsp. Olive oil

Directions:

1. On medium-high fire, place an ovenproof skillet and heat oil.

2. Pan Fry chicken for 3 to 5 minutes per side or until cooked through.

3. Pour marinara sauce, stir and continue cooking for 3 minutes.

4. Turn off fire, add mozzarella and breadcrumbs on top.

5. Pop into a preheated broiler on high and broil for 10 minutes or until breadcrumbs are browned, and mozzarella is melted.

6. Remove from broiler, serve and enjoy.

11.Chicken and White Bean

Total time: 1 hour 20 min

Prep time: 10 min

Cook time: 70 min

Yield: 6 servings

Ingredients:

- 2 tbsp. Fresh cilantro, chopped
- 2 cups grated low-fat Monterey jack cheese
- 3 cups water
- 1/8 tsp. Cayenne pepper
- 2 tsp. Pure Chile powder
- 2 tsp. ground cumin
- 1 4-oz can chop green chills
- 1 cup corn kernels
- 2 15-oz cans white beans, drained and rinsed
- 2 garlic cloves
- 1 medium onion, diced
- 2 tbsp. Extra virgin olive oil
- 1 lb. Chicken breasts, boneless and skinless

Directions:

1. Slice the chicken breasts into 1/2-inch chunks and season with salt and pepper.

2. Place a large anti-adhesive fry pan and heat oil on high fire.

3. Sauté the pieces of chicken for 3 to 4 minutes, or until finely browned.

4. Reduce the heat to mild and add the onion and garlic.

5. Cook for 5 to 6 minutes or until it is translucent with onions.

6. Stir in the sugar, peppers, chilies, maize, and beans. Just get it to a boil.

7. When baked, boil slowly and proceed to simmer for an hour, uncovered.

8. Garnish it with a dash of cilantro and a tablespoon of cheese to serve.

36. Chicken Pad Thai

Total time: 20 min

Prep time: 10 min

Cook time: 10 min

Yield: 6 servings

Ingredients:

- 2 medium sized carrots, julienned
- 1 12oz package broccoli slaw
- 5 green onions, chopped
- 5 tbsp. Fresh cilantro, chopped
- ½ tbsp. Coconut vinegar
- 4 tbsp. Fresh lime juice
- 1 tbsp. Coconut amines
- 3 tbsp. Fish sauce
- 5 cloves garlic, crushed
- 2 tbsp. Extra virgin coconut oil
- 1 ½ lb. Organic chicken meat, cut into chunks

Directions:

1. Over medium pressure, heat the skillet and apply the coconut oil.

2. For one minute, sauté the garlic and onion.

3. Add the chicken, then simmer for 5 minutes.

4. Placed the amines in the coconut, fish sauce, vinegar, and lime juice. Increase the heat and boil until the chicken is cooked thoroughly.

5. Add the carrots and broccoli slaw. Constantly stir until the vegetables become tender.

6. Garnish with green onions and cilantro.

12.Chicken Thighs with Butternut Squash

Total time: 40 min

Prep time: 10 min

Cook time: 30 min

Yield: 6 servings

Ingredients:

- 3 cups butternut squash, cubed

- 6 boneless chicken thighs

- A sprig of fresh sage, chopped

- 1 tbsp. Olive oil

- Salt and pepper to taste

Directions:

1. Preheat the 425°f oven.

2. Sauté the butternut squash in a skillet and season with salt and pepper to taste. Remove from the skillet after the squash is cooked and put aside.

3. Using the same pan, add oil and cook the chicken thighs on either side for 10 minutes.

4. Season with salt and pepper and return the squash to the mixture.

5. Take the skillet from the stove and cook it for 15 minutes in the oven.

6. Serving and enjoying!

13.Cajun Rice & Chicken

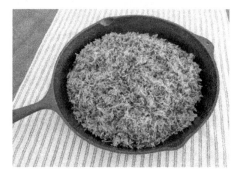

Total time: 30 min

Prep time: 10 min

Cook time: 20 min

Yield: 6 servings

Ingredients:

- 1 tablespoon oil
- 1 onion, diced
- 3 cloves of garlic, minced
- 1-pound chicken breasts, sliced
- 1 tablespoon Cajun seasoning
- 1 tablespoon tomato paste
- 3 cups chicken broth
- 1 ½ cups brown rice, rinsed
- 1 bell pepper, chopped

Directions:

1. Place a heavy-bottomed pot on medium-high fire and heat for 2 minutes.
2. Add oil and heat for a minute.
3. Sauté the onion and garlic until fragrant.

4. Stir in the chicken breasts and season with Cajun seasoning.

5. Continue cooking for 3 minutes.

6. Add the tomato paste, rice, and chicken broth. Bring to a boil while stirring to dissolve the tomato paste.

7. Once boiling, lower fire to a simmer, cover and cook until liquid is fully absorbed around 15 minutes.

8. Turn off the fire and let it stand for another 5 minutes before serving.

14.Vegetable Lover's Chicken Soup

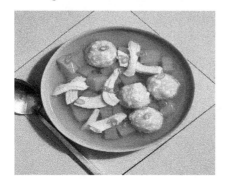

Total time: 30 min

Prep time: 10 min

Cook time: 20 min

Yield: 4 servings

Ingredients:

- 1 ½ cups baby spinach
- 2 tbsp. Orzo (tiny pasta)
- ¼ cup dry white wine
- 1 14oz low sodium chicken broth
- 2 plum tomatoes, chopped
- 1/8 tsp. Salt
- ½ tsp. Italian seasoning
- 1 large shallot, chopped
- 1 small zucchini, diced
- 8-oz chicken tenders
- 1 tbsp. Extra virgin olive oil

Directions:

1. In a large saucepan, heat oil over medium heat and add the chicken. Stir occasionally for 8 minutes until browned. Transfer in a plate. Set aside.

2. In the same saucepan, add the zucchini, Italian seasoning, shallot and salt and often stir until the vegetables are softened around 4 minutes.

3. Add the tomatoes, wine, broth and orzo and increase the heat to high to bring the mixture to boil. Reduce the heat and simmer.

4. Add the cooked chicken and stir in the spinach last.

5. Serve hot.

6.

15.Coconut Flour Cheesy Garlic Biscuits

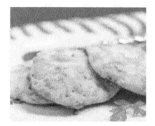

Total time: 20 min

Prep time: 10 min

Cook time: 10 min

Yield: 4 servings

Ingredients:

- 1/3 cup of coconut flour
- 1/2 teaspoon of baking powder
- 1/2 teaspoon of garlic powder
- 1 large egg
- 1/4 cup of unsalted butter, melted and divided
- 1/2 cup of shredded sharp Cheddar cheese
- 1 scallion, sliced

Directions:

1. In a broad dish, combine the coconut flour, baking powder, and garlic powder together.

2. Add the egg, half of the melted butter, the scallions and the cheddar cheese. In a 6 'circular baking tray, pour the mixture. Place it within the Air Fryer frame.

3. Set the temperature to 320 degrees F and change the 12-minute timer.

4. Remove and allow to cool fully from the pan to eat. Slice into four pieces and pour on any remaining butter.

16.Radish Chips

Total time: 20 min

Prep time: 10 min

Cook time: 10 min

Yield: 4 servings

Ingredients:

- 2 cups of water
- 1-pound of radishes
- 1/4 teaspoon of onion powder
- 1/4 teaspoon of paprika
- 1/2 teaspoon of garlic powder
- 2 tablespoons of coconut oil, melted

Directions:

1. Place water on a stovetop and bring to a boil in a medium saucepan.
2. Cut the top and bottom of each radish, then thinly and finely slice each radish with a mandolin. You could use the slicing blade in the food processor for this point, too.
3. Place the radish slices for 5 minutes in boiling water, or until they are translucent. To retain additional moisture, remove it from the bath and place it in a clean kitchen towel.
4. Place the radish chips with the remaining ingredients in a large bowl and season until completely coated with grease. Place the radish chips inside the Air Fryer basket.
5. Set the timer for 5 minutes and turn to 320° F.
6. Two or three times, shake a basket during the cooking process.

17.Flatbread

Total time: 20 min

Prep time: 10 min

Cook time: 10 min

Yield: 4 servings

Ingredients:

- 1 cup of shredded mozzarella cheese
- 1/4 cup of blanched finely ground almond flour
- 1 ounce of full-Fat: cream cheese, softened

Directions:

1. In a large, microwave-safe bowl, melt the mozzarella for 30 seconds. Stir in the almond flour until it is smooth, then apply the cream cheese. Continue to mix until the dough emerges, softly kneading it if necessary with wet hands.

2. "Break the dough into two parts and stretch to 1/4" thickness between two parchments. To fit the Air Fryer tray, cut another slice of parchment.

3. On your parchment and in the Air Fryer, place a slice of flatbread and work in two batches if appropriate.

4. Set the temperature to 320 degrees F and set a seven-minute timer.

5. Turn halfway through the cooking time on the flat-bread. Serve hot.

18. Avocado Fries

Total time: 20 min

Prep time: 10 min

Cook time: 10 min

Yield: 4 servings

Ingredients:

- 2 medium avocados
- 1-ounce of pork rinds, finely ground

Directions:

1. Cut out half the avocado from each one. Smash the fuselage. Gently cut the peel, then break the beef into 1/4-inch-thick slices.

2. In a medium cup, place the pork rinds and press each slice of avocado onto the pork rinds to cover them entirely.

3. Set the temperature to 350° F and set five minutes for the timer.

4. Serve it hot.

19.Pita-Style Chips

Total time: 20 min

Prep time: 10 min

Cook time: 10 min

Yield: 4 servings

Ingredients:

- 1 cup of shredded mozzarella cheese

- ½ ounce of pork rinds, finely ground

- ¼ cup of blanched finely ground almond flour

- 1 large egg

Directions:

1. In a large microwave and microwave dish, place the mozzarella for 30 seconds or until it has melted. Attach the remaining ingredients and stir to a smooth finish; the dough forms into a ball easily. If the dough is too hard, microwave it for 15 seconds.

2. Roll out the dough between two sheets of parchment into a large rectangle and then use a knife to cut triangle-shaped chips. Put the Air Fryer chips in the basket.

3. Set the temperature to 350° F and set five minutes for the timer.

4. The chips will be golden in color and sturdy when done. When they cool down, they'll be even firmer.

20.Roasted Eggplant

Total time: 20 min

Prep time: 10 min

Cook time: 10 min

Yield: 4 servings

Ingredients:

- 1 large eggplant
- 2 tablespoons of olive oil
- 1/4 teaspoon of salt
- 1/2 teaspoon of garlic powder

Directions:

1. Split the top and bottom of the eggplant. Break the eggplant into thick, thin strips.

2. Using olive oil to brush the slices and dust with salt and garlic powder. Place the bits in the jar with the eggplant.

3. Set the temperature to 390° F for 15 minutes and change the timer.

4. Serve promptly and enjoy yourself!

21.Parmesan-Herb Focaccia Bread

Total time: 20 min

Prep time: 10 min

Cook time: 10 min

Yield: 4 servings

Ingredients:

- 1 cup of shredded mozzarella cheese
- 1 ounce of full-Fat: cream cheese
- 1 cup of blanched finely ground almond flour
- 1/4 cup of ground golden flaxseed
- 1/4 cup of grated Parmesan cheese

- 1/2 teaspoon of baking soda

- 2large eggs

- 1/2 teaspoon of garlic powder

- 1/4 teaspoon of dried basil

- 1/4 teaspoon of dried rosemary

- 2 tablespoons of salted butter, melted and divided

Directions:

1. Place the mozzarella, cream cheese, and almond flour for 1 minute in a large microwave-safe bowl and microwave. Parmesan, flaxseed, and baking soda are added, and stir until the ball is smooth. If the mixture cools so fast, so it would be impossible to combine. When needed, return to the microwave to rewarm for 10-15 seconds.

2. The substitute ducks. To Mix them to the full, you can need to use your hands. Only keep frying, and then add them to the batter.

3. Mix the basil and rosemary with the powdered garlic dough and knead them into the dough. In a round baking pan, grease 1 tablespoon of melted butter. Similarly, put the dough in the pan. Place the pan in an Air Fryer basket.

4. Set the temperature to 400 degrees F and for 10 minutes, change the timer.

5. If the bread begins to get too black, cover with foil after 7 minutes.

6. Remove and cool for at least 30 minutes, then combine and eat with the remaining butter.

22.Quick and Easy Home Fries

Total time: 20 min

Prep time: 10 min

Cook time: 10 min

Yield: 4 servings

Ingredients:

- 1 medium jicama, peeled
- 1 tablespoon of coconut oil, melted
- 1/4 teaspoon of ground black pepper
- ½ teaspoon of pink Himalayan salt
- 1 medium green bell pepper, seeded and diced
- 1/2 medium white onion, peeled and diced

Directions:

1. Split the cubed jicama. Put it in a large bowl and mix until seasoned with coconut oil. Sprinkle with salt and pepper. Place the pepper and onion in a jar with the fryer.

2. Adjust the temperature and set a 10-minute timer to 400°F. Shake it three times before cooking it. Around the sides, Jicama will be smooth and dark and serve immediately.

23. Jicama Fries

Total time: 20 min

Prep time: 10 min

Cook time: 10 min

Yield: 4 servings

Ingredients:

- 1 small jicama, peeled
- 3/4 teaspoon of chili powder
- 1/4 teaspoon of garlic powder
- 1/4 teaspoon of onion powder
- 1/4 teaspoon of ground black pepper

Directions:

1. Break the jicama into cubes of 1'. Place in a large bowl and mix until coated with the coconut oil. Sprinkle with salt and pepper. In the fryer pan, put the pepper and onion.

2. Adjust the temperature and set a 10-minute timer to 400° F.

3. Shake two or three times before cooking. Jicama around the edges will be smooth and dark and will serve instantly.

24.Fried Green Tomatoes

Total time: 20 min

Prep time: 10 min

Cook time: 10 min

Yield: 4 servings

Ingredients:

- 2 medium green tomatoes
- 1 large egg
- 1/4 cup of blanched finely ground almond flour
- 1/3 cup of grated Parmesan cheese

Directions:

1. Break the tomatoes into 1/2-inch-thick slices. In a medium bowl, whisk the egg. In a large bowl, combine the almond flour and parmesan.

2. Dip each tomato slice into the egg, then dredge in the almond flour mixture and drop the slices in the basket of the Air Fryer.

3. Set the temperature to 400 degrees F and set a seven-minute timer.

4. Halfway through the duration of cooking, turn the slices. Serve immediately.

25.Fried Pickles

Total time: 20 min

Prep time: 10 min

Cook time: 10 min

Yield: 4 servings

Ingredients:

- 1 tablespoon of coconut flour
- 1/3 cup of blanched finely ground almond flour
- 1 teaspoon of chili powder
- 1/4 teaspoon of garlic powder
- 1 large egg
- 1 cup of sliced pickles

Directions:

1. In a medium dish, mix the coconut flour, almond meal, chili powder, and garlic powder.

2. Whisk the egg in a tiny mug.

3. Pat with a paper towel on each pickle and dunk in the egg. Then dredge in the mixture with flour. Put the pickles in the bowl for Air Fryer.

4. Switch to 400° F and set the timer for 5 minutes.

5. Flip the pickles halfway through the duration of preparation.

26.Pork and Potatoes

Preparation time: 5 minutes

Cooking time: 25 minutes

Servings: 4

Ingredients:

- 2 cups creamer potatoes, rinsed and dried
- 1 (1-pound) pork tenderloin, slice into 1-inch cubes
- 1 onion, red bell pepper, 2 garlic clover
- ½ teaspoon dried oregano
- 2 tablespoons low-sodium chicken broth

Directions:

1. To coat, toss the potatoes and olive oil.

2. Move the potatoes to the basket of an air fryer. For 15 minutes, bake.

3. Combine the bacon, cabbage, tomato, red bell pepper, garlic, and oregano together.

4. Drizzle the chicken broth with it. Place the bowl in the basket of an air fryer. During frying, roast and shake the basket once before the pork hits a meat thermometer of at least 145 ° f, and the potatoes are tender. Immediately serve.

27. Pork and Fruit Kebabs

Preparation time: 15 minutes

Cooking time: 9 to 12 minutes

Servings: 4

Ingredients:

- 1/3 cup apricot jam
- 2 tablespoons freshly squeezed lemon juice
- ½ teaspoon dried tarragon
- 1 (1-pound) pork tenderloin, slice into 1-inch cubes
- 4 plums, small apricots, pitted and halved

Directions:

1. Combine the jam, lemon juice, tarragon and olive oil.

2. To coat, add the pork and stir. Place it aside at room temperature for 10 minutes.

3. Thread the bacon, plums, and apricots onto 4 metal skewers that fit into the air fryer, alternating the items. Rub with a combination of any leftover jelly. Discard every marinade that exists.

4. In an air fryer, grill the kebabs for 9 to 12 minutes. Immediately serve.

28. Steak and Vegetable Kebabs

Preparation time: 15 minutes

Cooking time: 7 minutes

Servings: 4

Ingredients:

- 2 tablespoons balsamic vinegar
- ½ teaspoon dried marjoram
- ¾ pound round steak, cut into 1-inch pieces
- 1 cup red bell pepper, cherry tomatoes
- 16 button mushrooms

Directions:

1. Stir together the balsamic vinegar, olive oil, black pepper and marjoram.

2. To coat, add the steak and stir. Leave it to rest at room temperature for 9 minutes.

3. Thread the meat, red bell pepper, mushrooms and tomatoes onto 8 bamboo or metal skewers that match in the air fryer, rotating products.

4. Grill for 6 minutes in the air-fryer. Immediately serve.

29. Spicy Grilled Steak

Preparation time: 7 minutes

Cooking time: 9 minutes

Servings: 4

Ingredients:

- 2 tablespoons low-sodium salsa
- 1 tablespoon chipotle pepper, apple cider vinegar
- 1 teaspoon ground cumin
- 1/8 tsp. Red pepper flakes
- ¾ lb. Sirloin tip steak mildly pounded to about 1/3 inch thick

Directions:

1. Add chili, chipotle pepper, cider vinegar, cumin, black pepper and red pepper flakes. Scrub this mixture onto each steak piece on both sides. Let it stand at room temperature for 15 minutes.

2. In an air fryer, grill the steaks, two at a time, for 6 to 9 minutes.

3. To stay warm, put the steaks on a clean plate and cover them with aluminum foil. Repeat for the steaks that remain.

4. Thinly chop the steaks against the grain and serve.

30. Greek Vegetable Skillet
Preparation time: 10 minutes

Cooking time: 19 minutes

Servings: 4

Ingredients:

- ½ pound 96 percent lean ground beef
- 2 medium tomatoes, garlic clove
- 2 cups fresh baby spinach
- 1/3 cup low-sodium beef broth
- 2 tablespoons crumbled low-sodium feta cheese, lemon juice

Directions:

1. Crumble the beef in a 6-by-2-inch metal pan. Cook for 3 to 7 minutes in an air fryer, stirring once during frying until browned. Drain some fat or liquid out.

2. To the pan, add the tomatoes, 1 onion, and garlic. Air-fry for an additional 4 to 8 minutes.

3. Spinach, lemon juice, and beef broth are added. Air-fry for an additional 2 or 4 minutes.

4. Place the feta cheese on top of it and serve right away.

31. Light Herbed Meatballs
Preparation time: 10 minutes

Cooking time: 17 minutes

Servings: 24

Ingredients:

- 2 garlic cloves, minced

- 1 slice low-sodium whole-wheat bread, crumbled

- 3 tablespoons 1 percent milk

- 1 teaspoon dried marjoram, basil

- 1-pound 96 percent lean ground beef

Directions:

1. Combine the onion, garlic, and olive oil in a 6-by-2-inch pan. For 2 to 4 minutes, air-fry.

2. Put the vegetables in a medium bowl and combine with the bread crumbs, milk, basil, and marjoram. Mix thoroughly.

3. Add some ground beef. Run the mixture softly but thoroughly with your hands until mixed. Shape about 24 (1-inch) meatballs into a meat mixture.

4. Bake the meatballs, in lots, for 12 to 17 minutes in the air-fryer basket. Immediately serve.

32. Brown Rice and Beef-Stuffed Bell Peppers
Preparation time: 10 minutes

Cooking time: 16 minutes

Servings: 4

Ingredients:

- ½ cup grated carrot

- 1 cup cooked brown rice

- 1 cup chopped cooked low-sodium roast beef

- 4 bell peppers, 2 medium beefsteak tomatoes, onion

- 1 teaspoon dried marjoram

Directions:

1. Strip the bell pepper tops from the stems and chop the tops.

2. Combine the chopped bell pepper, onion, carrot, and olive oil in a 6-by-2-inch pan. Cook for 4 minutes, or until the vegetables are soft and crispy.

3. To a medium bowl, shift the vegetable. Add the onions, brown rice, marjoram, and roast beef. Stir to blend.

4. Stuff the combination of the vegetables into the bell peppers. Place the bell peppers in the basket of an air fryer. Bake or until the peppers are tender and the filling is sweet, for 14 minutes.

5. Instantly serve.

33.Beef and Broccoli

Preparation time: 10 minutes

Cooking time: 18 minutes

Servings: 4

Ingredients:

- ½ cup low-sodium beef broth

- 1 teaspoon low-sodium soy sauce

- 12 ounces sirloin strip steak, cut into 1-inch cubes

- 1 cup sliced cremini mushrooms, onion, ginger

- 2½ cups broccoli florets

Directions:

1. Stir 2 tablespoons of cornstarch, beef broth, and soy sauce together.

2. Attach the beef and cover with a toss. Set aside at room temperature for 5 minutes.

3. Move the beef from the broth combination into a small metal bowl with a slotted spoon.

4. Attach the beef to the broccoli, cabbage, mushrooms, and ginger. Place the bowl in the air fryer and cook for 12 to 15 minutes or on a meat thermometer until the beef hits at least 145 ° f and the vegetables are tender.

5. Attach the reserved broth and simmer for another 2 to 3 minutes or until the sauce is ready to boil.

6. If needed, serve immediately over hot cooked brown rice.

34.Beef and Fruit Stir-Fry

Preparation time: 15 minutes

Cooking time: 11 minutes

Servings: 4

Ingredients:

- 12 ounces sirloin tip steak, thinly sliced
- 1 tablespoon lime juice, cornstarch
- 1 cup canned mandarin orange segments, pineapple chunks
- 1 teaspoon low-sodium soy sauce
- 2 scallions, white and green parts, sliced

Directions:

1. Mix the lime juice with the steak. Just put aside.

2. Combine 3 tablespoons of reserved orange mandarin juice, 3 tablespoons of reserved pineapple juice, soy sauce, and cornstarch thoroughly.

3. Dry the beef and place it in a medium-sized metal cup, reserving the juice. Stir the reserved juice into the mixture of the mandarin-pineapple juice. And put aside.

4. Add to the steak the olive oil and the scallions. Put the metal bowl in the air fryer and reheat for 3 to 4 minutes, or shake the basket once during the cooking, until the steak is almost cooked.

5. Stir in a blend of mandarin oranges, pineapple and milk. Cook for 3 to 7 more minutes, or until the sauce is bubbling and the beef on a meat thermometer is soft and reaches at least 145 ° f.

6. If needed, stir and serve over warm fried brown rice.

35.Perfect Garlic Butter Steak
Preparation time: 20 minutes

Cooking time: 12 minutes

Servings: 4

Ingredients:

- 2 rib-eye steaks

- Garlic butter:

- ½ cup softened butter

- 2 tbsp. Chopped fresh parsley

- 2 garlic cloves, minced

- 1 tsp. Worcestershire sauce

Directions:

1. Add each of the ingredients together to prepare the garlic butter.

2. Place the document on parchment. Roll it up and put it in the refrigerator.

3. Just let steaks remain at room temperature for 20 minutes.

4. Brush some of the grease, salt, and pepper with it.

5. Pre-heat up to 400 ° f (200 ° c) with your hot air fryer.

6. 12 minutes to cook, rotating halfway through the cooking process. Just serve.

7. Top the steaks with the garlic butter and let hang for 5 minutes.

8. Enjoy and Serve!

36.Crispy Pork Medallions

Preparation time: 20 minutes

Cooking time: 5 minutes

Servings: 2

Ingredients:

- 1 pork loin, 330 g, cut into 6 or 7 slices of 4 cm

- Asian marinade:

- 1 tsp. Salt reduced tamari sauce, olive oil

- 1 clementine juice

- 1 pinch cayenne pepper

- 2 cloves garlic, pressed

Directions:

1. Get the marinade prepared first. Combine all the ingredients in a dish. Salt the medallions gently, apply pepper and sprinkle with 1 tsp. About paprika. Place these in the marinade and turn them to soak them full many times. Cover with plastic wrap and marinate at room temperature for 1 hour.

2. Merge 1/3 of a cup of breadcrumbs, 1/2 of orange zest and 2 grams of parmesan cheese in a deep dish to prepare the covering.

3. Remove the marinade medallions and dry them on absorbent paper after the time for maceration has expired. Fill with mustard, and move on to the sheet that is crunchy. Lightly brush with oil.

4. Heat the air-fryer to 350 degrees F. Place the medallions in the basket with the fryer. Cook for five minutes, stir, and then bring it back in the fryer for another minute. Immediately serve.

37.Parmesan Meatballs

Preparation time: 10 minutes

Cooking time: 20 minutes

Servings: 6

Ingredients:

- 2 lbs. Ground beef
- 2 eggs
- 1 cup ricotta cheese
- 1/4 cup parmesan cheese shredded
- 1/2 cup panko breadcrumbs
- 1/4 cup basil chopped
- 1/4 cup parsley chopped
- 1 tablespoon fresh oregano chopped
- 2 teaspoon kosher salt
- 1 teaspoon ground fennel
- 1/2 teaspoon red pepper flakes
- 32 oz. spaghetti sauce, to serve

Directions:

1. In a bowl, carefully mix the beef with all the other meatball ingredients.

2. Create tiny meatballs out of this combination, then put them in the basket of the air fryer.

3. Click the Air Fry Oven control button and switch the knob to pick the bake mode.

4. To set the cooking time to 20 minutes, click the time button and change the dial once again.

5. Now press the temp button to set the temperature at 400 degrees f and rotate the dial.

6. When preheated, put the basket of meatballs in the oven and close the lid.

7. When baked, turn the meatballs halfway through and then start cooking.

8. On top, pour the spaghetti sauce.

9. Serve it hot.

38.Tricolor Beef Skewers

Preparation time: 10 minutes

Cooking time: 25 minutes

Servings: 4

Ingredients:

- 3 garlic cloves, minced
- 4 tablespoon rapeseed oil
- 1 cup cottage cheese, cubed
- 16 cherry tomatoes
- 2 tablespoon cider vinegar
- Large bunch thyme
- 1 ¼ lb. Boneless beef, diced

Directions:

1. Toss beef with all its thyme, oil, vinegar, and garlic.

2. Marinate the thyme beef for 2 hours in a closed container in the refrigerator.

3. Thread the marinated beef, cheese, and tomatoes on the skewers.

4. Place these skewers in an air fryer basket.

5. Press the "power button" of the air fry oven and turn the dial to select the "air fry" mode.

6. Press the time button and again turn the dial to set the cooking time to 25 minutes.

7. Now push the temp button and rotate the dial to set the temperature at 350 degrees f.

8. Once preheated, place the air fryer basket in the oven and close its lid.

9. Flip the skewers when cooked halfway through, then resume cooking.

10. Serve warm.

39. Yogurt Beef Kebabs

Preparation time: 10 minutes

Cooking time: 25 minutes

Servings: 4

Ingredients:

- ½ cup yogurt
- 1½ tablespoon mint
- 1 teaspoon ground cumin
- 1 cup eggplant, diced
- 10.5 oz. Lean beef, diced
- ½ small onion, cubed

Directions:

1. Whisk yogurt with mint and cumin in a suitable bowl.

2. Toss in beef cubes and mix well to coat. Marinate for 30 minutes.

3. Alternatively, thread the beef, onion, and eggplant on the skewers.

4. Place these beef skewers in the air fry basket.

5. Press the "power button" of the air fry oven and turn the dial to select the "air fryer" mode.

6. Press the time button and again turn the dial to set the cooking time to 25 minutes.

7. Now push the temp button and rotate the dial to set the temperature at 370 degrees f.

8. Once preheated, place the air fryer basket in the oven and close its lid.

9. Flip the skewers when cooked halfway through, then resume cooking.

10. Serve warm.

40.Agave Beef Kebabs

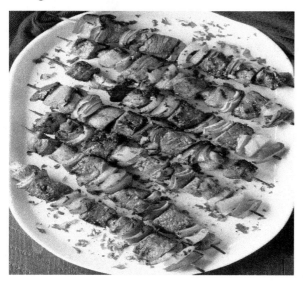

Preparation time: 10 minutes

Cooking time: 20 minutes

Servings: 6

Ingredients:

- 2 lbs. Beef steaks, cubed
- Two tablespoon jerk seasoning
- Zest and juice of 1 lime
- 1 tablespoon agave syrup
- ½ teaspoon thyme leaves, chopped

Directions:

1. Mix beef with jerk seasoning, lime juice, zest, agave and thyme.

2. Toss well to coat, then marinate for 30 minutes.

3. Alternatively, thread the beef on the skewers.

4. Place these beef skewers in the air fry basket.

5. Press the "power button" of the air fry oven and turn the dial to select the "air fryer" mode.

6. Press the time button and again turn the dial to set the cooking time to 20 minutes.

7. Now push the temp button and rotate the dial to set the temperature at 360 degrees f.

8. Once preheated, place the air fryer basket in the oven and close its lid.

9. Flip the skewers when cooked halfway through, then resume cooking.

10. Serve warm.

41.Beef Skewers with Potato Salad

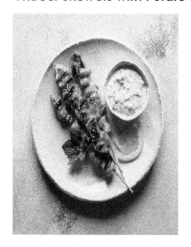

Preparation time: 10 minutes

Cooking time: 25 minutes

Servings: 4

Ingredients:

- Juice ½ lemon
- 2 tablespoon olive oil
- 1 garlic clove, crushed
- 1 ¼ lb. Diced beef
- For the salad
- 2 potatoes, boiled, peeled and diced
- 4 large tomatoes, chopped
- 1 cucumber, chopped
- 1 handful black olives, chopped
- 9 oz. Pack feta cheese, crumbled
- 1 bunch of mint, chopped

Directions:

1. Whisk lemon juice with garlic and olive oil in a bowl.

2. Toss in beef cubes and mix well to coat. Marinate for 30 minutes.

3. Alternatively, thread the beef on the skewers.

4. Place these beef skewers in the air fry basket.

5. Press the "power button" of the air fry oven and turn the dial to select the "air fryer" mode.

17. Press the time button and again turn the dial to set the cooking time to 25 minutes.

18. Now push the temp button and rotate the dial to set the temperature at 360 degrees f.

19. Once preheated, place the air fryer basket in the oven and close its lid.

20. Flip the skewers when cooked halfway through, then resume cooking.

21. Meanwhile, whisk all the salad ingredients in a salad bowl.

22. Serve the skewers with prepared salad.

42. Classic Souvlaki Kebobs

Preparation time: 10 minutes

Cooking time: 20 minutes

Servings: 6

Ingredients:

- 2 ¼ lbs. Beef shoulder fat trimmed, cut into chunks
- 1/3 cup olive oil
- ½ cup red wine
- 2 teaspoon dried oregano
- ½ cup of orange juice
- 1 teaspoon orange zest
- 2 garlic cloves, crushed

Directions:

1. Whisk olive oil, red wine, oregano, oranges juice, zest, and garlic in a suitable bowl.

2. Toss in beef cubes and mix well to coat. Marinate for 30 minutes.

3. Alternatively, thread the beef, onion, and bread on the skewers.

4. Place these beef skewers in the air fry basket.

5. Press the "power button" of the air fry oven and turn the dial to select the "air fryer" mode.

6. Press the time button and again turn the dial to set the cooking time to 20 minutes.

7. Now push the temp button and rotate the dial to set the temperature at 370 degrees f.

8. Once preheated, place the air fryer basket in the oven and close its lid.

9. Flip the skewers when cooked halfway through, then resume cooking.

10. Serve warm.

43. Harissa Dipped Beef Skewers

Preparation time: 10 minutes

Cooking time: 16 minutes

Servings: 6

Ingredients:

- 1 lb. Beef mince
- 4 tablespoon harissa
- 2 oz. Feta cheese
- One large red onion, shredded
- 1 handful parsley, chopped
- 1 handful mint, chopped
- 1 tablespoon olive oil
- Juice 1 lemon

Directions:

1. Whisk the lean beef in a bowl of harissa, onion, feta, and seasoning.

2. From this mixture, make 12 sausages, then thread them onto the skewers.

3. In the air-fry basket, put these beef skewers.

4. Click the Air Fry Oven control button and switch the knob to pick the bake mode.

5. To set the cooking time to 16 minutes, press the time button and turn the knob over again.

6. Now press the temp button to set the temperature at 370 degrees f and rotate the dial.

7. Place the air fryer basket in the oven until pre-heated and close the lid.

8. When done, rotate the skewers halfway through and then start cooking.

9. In a salad bowl, toss the remaining salad ingredients together.

10. Using tomato salad to eat beef skewers.

44. Onion Pepper Beef Kebobs

Preparation time: 10 minutes

Cooking time: 20 minutes

Servings: 4

Ingredients:

- 2 tablespoon pesto paste
- 2/3 lb. Beefsteak, diced
- 2 red peppers, cut into chunks
- 2 red onions, cut into wedges
- 1 tablespoon olive oil

Directions:

1. Toss the harissa and oil into the beef balls, then blend well to coat. For 30 minutes, marinate.

2. Thread the beef, onion, and peppers on the skewers as an option.

3. In the air-fry basket, put these beef skewers.

4. Click the air fryer's "power button" and change the knob to choose "air fryer" mode.

5. To set the cooking time to 20 minutes, click the time button and change the dial once again.

6. Now press the temp button to set the temperature at 370 degrees f and rotate the dial.

7. Place the air fryer basket in the oven until pre-heated and close the lid.

8. When done, rotate the skewers halfway through and then start cooking.

9. Serve it hot.

45.Mayo Spiced Kebobs

Preparation time: 10 minutes

Cooking time: 10 minutes

Servings: 4

Ingredients:

- 2 tablespoon cumin seed
- 2 tablespoon coriander seed
- 2 tablespoon fennel seed
- 1 tablespoon paprika
- 2 tablespoon garlic mayonnaise
- 4 garlic cloves, finely minced
- ½ teaspoon ground cinnamon
- 1 ½ lb. Lean minced beef

Directions:

1. Blend all the spices and seeds with garlic, cream, and cinnamon in a blender.

2. Add this cream paste to the minced beef, then mix well.

3. Make 8 sausages and thread each on the skewers.

4. Place these beef skewers in the air fry basket.

5. Press the "power button" of the air fry oven and turn the dial to select the "air fryer" mode.

6. Press the time button and again turn the dial to set the cooking time to 10 minutes.

7. Now push the temp button and rotate the dial to set the temperature at 370 degrees f.

8. Once preheated, place the air fryer basket in the oven and close its lid.

9. Flip the skewers when cooked halfway through, then resume cooking.

10. Serve warm.

46.Beef with Orzo Salad

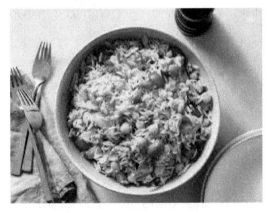

Preparation time: 10 minutes

Cooking time: 27 minutes

Servings: 4

Ingredients:

- 2/3 lbs. Beef shoulder, cubed
- 1 teaspoon ground cumin
- ½ teaspoon cayenne pepper
- 1 teaspoon sweet smoked paprika
- 1 tablespoon olive oil
- 24 cherry tomatoes
- Salad:
- ½ cup orzo, boiled
- ½ cup frozen pea
- 1 large carrot, grated
- Small pack coriander, chopped
- Small pack mint, chopped
- Juice 1 lemon
- 2 tablespoon olive oil

Directions:

1. Toss tomatoes and beef with oil, paprika, pepper, and cumin in a bowl.
2. Alternatively, thread the beef and tomatoes on the skewers.
3. Place these beef skewers in the air fry basket.
4. Press the "power button" of the air fry oven and turn the dial to select the "air fryer" mode.
5. Press the time button and again turn the dial to set the cooking time to 25 minutes.
6. Now push the temp button and rotate the dial to set the temperature at 370 degrees f.
7. Once preheated, place the air fryer basket in the oven and close its lid.

8. Flip the skewers when cooked halfway through, then resume cooking.

9. Meanwhile, sauté carrots and peas with olive oil in a pan for 2 minutes.

10. Stir in mint, lemon juice, coriander, and cooked couscous.

11. Serve skewers with the couscous salad.

47.Beef Zucchini Shashliks

Preparation time: 10 minutes

Cooking time: 25 minutes

Servings: 4

Ingredients:

- 1lb. Beef, boned and diced
- 1 lime, juiced and chopped
- 3 tablespoon olive oil
- 20 garlic cloves, chopped
- 1 handful rosemary, chopped
- 3 green peppers, cubed
- 2 zucchinis, cubed
- 2 red onions, cut into wedges

Directions:

1. Toss the beef with the rest of the skewer's ingredients in a bowl.

2. Thread the beef, peppers, zucchini, and onion on the skewers.

3. Place these beef skewers in the air fry basket.

4. Press the "power button" of the air fry oven and turn the dial to select the "air fryer" mode.

5. Press the time button and again turn the dial to set the cooking time to 25 minutes.

6. Now push the temp button and rotate the dial to set the temperature at 370 degrees f.

7. Once preheated, place the air fryer basket in the oven and close its lid.

8. Flip the skewers when cooked halfway through, then resume cooking.

9. Serve warm.

48. Delicious Zucchini Mix

Total time: 25 min

Prep time: 10 min

Cook time: 15 min

Yield: 6 servings

Ingredients:

- 6 zucchinis, halved and then sliced
- Salt and black pepper to the taste
- 1 tablespoon of butter
- 1 teaspoon of oregano, dried
- ½ cup yellow onion, chopped
- 3 garlic cloves, minced
- 2 ounces of parmesan, grated
- ¾ cup of heavy cream

Directions:

1. On medium-high prepare, heat a saucepan that suits the butter of your Air Fryer, add onion, stir and cook for 4 minutes.

2. Mix the garlic, zucchini, oregano, salt, pepper and heavy cream together, shake, fry in the air and boil at 350 degrees F for 10 minutes.

3. Stir in the parmesan cheese, whisk, split and eat.

49. Swiss Chard and Sausage

Total time: 30 min

Prep time: 10 min

Cook time: 25 min

Yield: 8 servings

Ingredients:

- 8 cups of Swiss chard, chopped
- ½ cup of onion, chopped
- 1 tablespoon of olive oil
- 1 garlic clove, minced
- Salt and black pepper to the taste
- 3 eggs
- 2 cups of ricotta cheese
- 1 cup of mozzarella, shredded
- A pinch of nutmeg
- ¼ cup of parmesan, grated
- 1-pound sausage, chopped

Directions:

1. Heat up the Air Fryer with a saucepan that suits the oil over medium heat, add onions, garlic, Swiss chard, salt, pepper and nutmeg, stir, cook and turn off for 2 minutes.

2. In a bowl of mozzarella, parmesan, ricotta, whisk the eggs, stir, spillover Swiss chard blend, shake, put in your Air Fryer and cook at 320 °F for 17 minutes.

3. Divide and consume between bowls.

50.Swiss Chard Salad

Total time: 18 min

Prep time: 5 min

Cook time: 10 min

Yield: 4 servings

Ingredients:

- 1 bunch of Swiss chard, torn
- 2 tablespoons of olive oil
- 1 small yellow onion, chopped
- A pinch of red pepper flakes
- ¼ cup of pine nuts, toasted
- ¼ cup of raisins
- 1 tablespoon of balsamic vinegar
- Salt and black pepper to the taste

Directions:

1. Heat a medium-hot saucepan that fits the oil with your Air Fryer, add the chard and onions, stir and cook for 5 minutes.
2. Add the salt, pepper, pepper flakes, raisins, pine nuts and vinegar, stir, fry and simmer at 350 degrees F. for 8 minutes.
3. Divide and consume between bowls.

51.Spanish Greens

Total time: 18 min

Prep time: 5 min

Cook time: 10 min

Yield: 4 servings

Ingredients:

- 1 apple, cored and chopped
- 1 yellow onion, sliced
- 3 tablespoons of olive oil
- ¼ cup of raisins
- 6 garlic cloves, chopped
- ¼ cup of pine nuts, toasted
- ¼ cup of balsamic vinegar
- 5 cups of mixed spinach and chard

- Salt and black pepper to the taste
- A pinch of nutmeg

Directions:

1. Over medium-high pressure, heat a saucepan that fits the oil with your Air Fryer, add onion, stir and cook for 3 minutes.

2. Add the onion, ginger, raisins, sugar, mixed spinach, chard, nutmeg, salt and pepper, stir, and roast for 5 minutes at 350 degrees F.

3. Brush on top, break into bowls and serve with pine nuts.

52. Flavored Air Fried Tomatoes

Total time: 25 min

Prep time: 10 min

Cook time: 15 min

Yield: 6 servings

Ingredients:

- 1 jalapeno pepper, chopped
- 4 garlic cloves, minced
- 2 pounds of cherry tomatoes, halved
- Salt and black pepper to the taste
- ¼ cup of olive oil
- ½ teaspoon of oregano, dried
- ¼ cup of basil, chopped
- ½ cup of parmesan, grated

Directions:

1. In a cup, add the tomatoes with garlic, jalapeno, season with salt, pepper and oregano, drizzle with the oil, blend to cover, put in your Air Fryer and cook at 380 °F for 15 minutes.

2. Move the tomatoes to a pan, add the basil and parmesan, toss and eat.

53.Italian Eggplant Stew

Total time: 25 min

Prep time: 10 min

Cook time: 15 min

Yield: 6 servings

Ingredients:

- 1 red onion, chopped
- 2 garlic cloves, chopped
- 1 bunch of parsley, chopped
- Salt and black pepper to the taste
- 1 teaspoon of oregano, dried
- 2 eggplants, cut into medium chunks
- 2 tablespoons of olive oil
- 2 tablespoons of capers, chopped
- 1 handful green olives, pitted and sliced
- 5 tomatoes, chopped
- 3 tablespoons of herb vinegar

Directions:

1. Heat a medium-hot saucepan that fits the oil of your Air Fryer, add the eggplant, oregano, salt, and pepper, stir and cook for 5 minutes.
2. Combine the garlic, onions, parsley, capers, olives, vinegar and tomatoes, stir, fry and prepare at 360 °F for 15 minutes.
3. Break and serve in pots.

54.Rutabaga and Cherry Tomatoes Mix

Total time: 25 min

Prep time: 10 min

Cook time: 15 min

Yield: 6 servings

Ingredients:

- 1 tablespoon of shallot, chopped
- 1 garlic clove, minced
- ¾ cup of cashews, soaked for a couple of hours and drained
- 2 tablespoons of nutritional yeast
- ½ cup of veggie stock
- Salt and black pepper to the taste
- 2 teaspoons of lemon juice

For the pasta:

- 1 cup of cherry tomatoes, halved
- 5 teaspoons of olive oil
- ¼ teaspoon of garlic powder
- 2 rutabagas, peeled and cut into thick noodles

Directions:

1. Heat a medium-hot saucepan that fits the oil of your Air Fryer, add the eggplant, oregano, salt, and pepper, stir and cook for 5 minutes.
2. Combine the garlic, onions, parsley, capers, olives, vinegar and tomatoes, stir, fry and prepare at 360 °F for 15 minutes.
3. Break and serve in pots.

55. Garlic Tomatoes

Total time: 25 min

Prep time: 10 min

Cook time: 15 min

Yield: 6 servings

Ingredients:

- 4 garlic cloves, crushed

- 1-pound mixed cherry tomatoes
- 3 thyme springs, chopped
- Salt and black pepper to the taste
- ¼ cup of olive oil

Directions:

1. In a bowl of salt, black pepper, garlic, olive oil and thyme, mix the tomatoes, brush, place in the Air Fryer, and cook at 360 °F for 15 minutes.

2. Divide the tomatoes into bowls and serve.

56.Tomato and Basil Tart

Total time: 25 min

Prep time: 10 min

Cook time: 15 min

Yield: 6 servings

Ingredients:

- 1 bunch of basil, chopped
- 4 eggs
- 1 garlic clove, minced
- Salt and black pepper to the taste
- ½ cup of cherry tomatoes halved
- ¼ cup of cheddar cheese, grated

Directions:

1. In a cup, combine the eggs with the cinnamon, black pepper, cheese and basil, then whisk together well.

2. Place the tomatoes on top, put in the fryer, and cook at 320 ° F for 14 minutes in a baking dish that fits with your Air Fryer.

3. Cut on and serve.

57.Zucchini Noodles Delight

Total time: 30 min

Prep time: 10 min

Cook time: 25 min

Yield: 6 servings

Ingredients:

- 2 tablespoons of olive oil
- 3 zucchinis, cut with a spiralizer
- 16 ounces of mushrooms, sliced
- ¼ cup sun-dried tomatoes, chopped
- 1 teaspoon of garlic, minced
- ½ cup of cherry tomatoes halved
- 2 cups of tomatoes sauce
- 2 cups of spinach, torn
- Salt and black pepper to the taste
- A bunch of basil, chopped

Directions:

1. In a bowl, place the zucchini noodles, season with salt and black pepper and leave for about 10 minutes.
2. Over medium-high heat, heat a pan that matches the oil with your Air Fryer, add the garlic, stir and cook for 1 minute.
3. Stir in mushrooms, sun-dried tomatoes, cherry tomatoes, spinach, cayenne, sauce, zucchini noodles, place in the Air Fryer, and cook at 320 degrees F for 10 minutes.
4. With sprinkled basil, divide between plates and pour-over.

58.Simple Tomatoes and Bell Pepper Sauce

Total time: 25 min

Prep time: 10 min

Cook time: 15 min

Yield: 6 servings

Ingredients:

- 2 red bell peppers, chopped
- 2 garlic cloves, minced
- 1-pound cherry tomatoes halved
- 1 teaspoon of rosemary, dried
- 3 bay leaves
- 2 tablespoons of olive oil
- 1 tablespoon of balsamic vinegar
- Salt and black pepper to the taste

Directions:

1. In a bowl, mix the tomatoes with the garlic, the salt, the black pepper, the rosemary, the bay leaves, half the oil, half the vinegar, and brush, and place in the Air Fryer and cook at 320 degrees F. for 15 minutes.

2. Meanwhile, in your food processor, mix the bell peppers with a touch of sea salt, black pepper, the rest of the oil, and the rest of the vinegar and mix very well.

3. Divide the roasted tomatoes into bowls, sauce them with the bell peppers and eat them.

59.Salmon with Thyme & Mustard

Preparation Time: 10 Minutes

Cooking Time: 10 Minutes

Servings: 2

Ingredients:

- 2 salmon fillets
- Salt and pepper to taste
- ½ teaspoon dried thyme
- 2 tablespoons mustard

- 2 teaspoons olive oil
- 1 clove garlic, minced
- 1 tablespoon brown sugar

Directions:

1. Sprinkle salt and pepper on both sides of the salmon.

2. In a bowl, combine the remaining ingredients.

3. Spread this mixture on top of the salmon.

4. Place the salmon in the air fryer.

5. Choose the air fry function.

6. Cook at 400 degrees F for 10 minutes.

60.Lemon Garlic Fish Fillet

Preparation Time: 10 Minutes

Cooking Time: 30 Minutes

Servings: 2-4

Ingredients:

- 2 white fish fillets
- Cooking spray
- ½ teaspoon lemon pepper
- ½ teaspoon garlic powder
- Salt and pepper to taste
- 2 teaspoon lemon juice

Directions:

1. Choose a bake setting in your air fryer oven.

2. Preheat it to 360 degrees F.

3. Spray fish fillets with oil.

4. Season fish fillets with lemon pepper, garlic powder, salt and pepper.

5. Add to the air fryer.

6. Cook at 360 degrees F for 20 minutes.

7. Drizzle with lemon juice.

61.Blackened Tilapia

Preparation Time: 10 Minutes

Cooking Time: 35 Minutes

Servings: 4

Ingredients:

- 4 tilapia fillets
- Cooking spray
- 2 teaspoons brown sugar
- 2 tablespoons paprika
- ¼ teaspoon cayenne pepper
- 1 teaspoon garlic powder
- 1 teaspoon dried oregano
- ½ teaspoon cumin
- Salt to taste

Directions:

1. Spray fish fillets with oil.

2. Mix the remaining ingredients in a bowl.

3. Sprinkle both sides of fish with spice mixture.

4. Add to the air fryer.

5. Set it to air fry.

6. Cook at 400 degrees F for 4 to 5 minutes per side.

62.Fish & Sweet Potato Chips

Preparation Time: 10 Minutes

Cooking Time: 35 Minutes

Servings: 4

Ingredients:

- 4 cups sweet potatoes, sliced into strips
- 1 teaspoon olive oil
- 1 egg, beaten
- 2/3 cup breadcrumbs
- 1 teaspoon lemon zest
- 2 fish fillets, sliced into strips
- ½ cup Greek yogurt
- 1 tablespoon shallots, chopped
- 1 tablespoon chives, chopped
- 2 teaspoons dill, chopped

Directions:

1. Toss in the oil with the sweet potatoes.

2. Cook in an air fryer for 10 minutes or until crispy at 360 degrees F.

3. Just put aside.

4. Dip the fish fillet into your egg.

5. Dredge with lemon zest mixed with breadcrumbs.

6. Fry for 12 minutes at 360 degrees F.

7. Mix the milk along with the remaining ingredients.

8. Serve with fish, sweet potato chips, and sauce.

63. Brussels Sprout Chips

Preparation Time: 10 Minutes

Cooking Time: 15 Minutes

Servings: 2

Ingredients:

- 2 cups Brussels sprouts, sliced thinly
- 1 tablespoon olive oil

- 1 teaspoon garlic powder
- Salt and pepper to taste
- 2 tablespoons Parmesan cheese, grated

Directions:

1. In the oil, throw the Brussels sprouts.

2. Sprinkle the garlic, salt, pepper and Parmesan cheese with the garlic powder.

3. Select the Bake function.

4. In an air fryer, add the Brussels sprouts.

5. Cook for 8 minutes at 350 degrees F.

6. Flip and cook for an additional 7 minutes.

64.Shrimp Spring Rolls with Sweet Chili Sauce

Preparation Time: 10 Minutes

Cooking Time: 30 Minutes

Servings: 4

Ingredients:

- 2 ½ tbsp... sesame oil, divided
- 1 cup julienne-cut red bell pepper
- 1 cup matchstick carrots
- 2 cups pre-shredded cabbage
- ¼ cup chopped fresh cilantro
- 2 tsp. fish sauce
- ¼ tsp. crushed red pepper
- 1 tbsp... fresh lime juice
- ¾ cup julienne-cut snow peas
- 4 oz. peeled, deveined raw shrimp, chopped
- 8 (8-inch-square) spring roll wrappers
- ½ cup sweet chili sauce

Directions:

1. Pour in 1.5 teaspoons of the oil and let it heat over high heat until it smokes slightly. Get a big skillet. Toss the bell pepper, carrots, and cabbage in it now. Allow it to cook until the mixture is lightly wilted when constantly stirring (this takes 1 or 1.5 minutes). Spread on a rimmed baking sheet and leave for 5 minutes to cool.

2. Combine the cilantro, fish sauce, crushed red pepper, lime juice, snow peas, crabs, and a mixture of cabbage in a large bowl. Lightly stir.

3. Place on the work surface the spring roll wrappers so that you are facing one corner. Shift 1/4 cup of filling into the center of each spring roll wrapper using your spoon, while spreading it from left to right and into a 3-inch-long strip.

4. While tucking the tip of the corner under the filling, fold the bottom corner of each wrapper over the filling. Fold the left and right corners over the filling. Using water, lightly brush the remaining corner and roll the filled end of the wrapper into the remaining corner. Lastly, click to close softly. Dust two teaspoons of oil with the unused spring rolls.

5. In the air fryer basket, transfer the first four spring rolls and allow them to cook at 390 ° F for about 7 minutes. Flip the spring rolls after the first five minutes. For the other spring rolls, do the same.

6. Serve alongside spicy beef sauce with the cooked spring rolls.

65.Coconut Shrimp and Apricot

Preparation Time: 5 Minutes

Cooking Time: 35 Minutes

Servings: 6

Ingredients:

- 1-1/2 lbs. large shrimp, uncooked
- 1-1/2 cups sweetened shredded coconut
- ½ cup panko bread crumbs
- 4 large egg whites
- ¼ tsp. salt

- ¼ tsp. ground black pepper
- 3 dashes Louisiana-style hot sauce
- ½ cup all-purpose flour
- Cooking spray

Sauce:

- 1 cup apricot preserves
- ¼ tsp. crushed red pepper flakes
- 1 tsp. cider vinegar

Directions:

1. Make sure the air fryer is preheated to 375 F.

2. Peel the shrimp, eliminate the veins, but leave the tails.

3. Pick a shallow bowl and combine the coconut and breadcrumbs together.

4. Whisk the egg whites, salt, pepper, and hot sauce into another small mug.

5. Take up a third small bowl and place the flour in it.

6. To lightly coat, dip the shrimp into the flour. Through shaking, remove any excess flour.

7. In the egg white mixture and then in the coconut mixture, dip the flour-coated shrimp. Pat to ensure the compliance of the coating.

8. Spray the basket with cooking spray in your air fryer. If required, you can work in batches.

9. In the air fryer basket, arrange the shrimps so that they form a single plate.

10. Allow them to cook for 4 minutes. Turn the shrimp to the other side and cook until the coconut is finely browned and the shrimp is pink (this takes about 4 minutes).

11. Take a small saucepan when cooking the shrimps and mix the sauce ingredients in it. Then cook and whisk the mixture until the preserves are melted over medium-low heat.

12. Alongside the freshly cooked shrimps, serve the sauce.

66.Coconut Shrimp and Lime Juice

Preparation Time: 5 Minutes

Cooking Time: 30 Minutes

Servings: 4

Ingredients:

- 1½ tsp. black pepper
- ½ cup all-purpose flour
- 2 large eggs
- 2/3 cup unsweetened flaked coconut
- 1/3 cup panko (Japanese-style breadcrumbs)
- 12 oz. medium peeled, deveined raw shrimp, tail-on (about 24 shrimp)
- Cooking spray
- ½ tsp. kosher salt

Sauce:

- ¼ cup lime juice
- 1 serrano chile, thinly sliced
- ¼ cup honey
- 2 tsp. chopped fresh cilantro (optional)

Directions:

1. Get a shallow dish – and make a mixture of the pepper and the flour.

2. In a second shallow dish, beat the eggs.

3. Get a third shallow dish and mix the coconut and panko in it.

4. Hold each shrimp by the tail and dip into the flour mixture without coating the tail. Shake to get rid of the excess flour.

5. Dip in the egg mixture and allow any excess to drip off.

6. Finally, dip in the coconut mixture and press to ensure adherence.

7. Coat the shrimp generously with the cooking spray.

8. Transfer half of the shrimp to the air fryer basket and allow to cook for 6 to 8 minutes at 400 F.

9. Halfway into cooking, turn the shrimp to the other side and season with ¼ teaspoon of the salt.

10. Do the same for the other shrimps and salt also.

11. In the meantime, get a small bowl and whisk the lime juice, Serrano chile, and honey together.

12. Sprinkle the cooked shrimp with cilantro, and serve alongside the sauce (if desired).

67.Lemon Pepper Shrimp

Preparation Time: 5 Minutes

Cooking Time: 20 Minutes

Servings: 2

Ingredients:

- 1 lemon, juiced
- ¼ tsp. paprika
- ¼ tsp. garlic powder
- 1 tsp. lemon pepper
- 1 tbsp... olive oil
- 12 oz. uncooked medium shrimp, peeled and deveined
- 1 lemon, sliced

Directions:

1. Ensure that your air fryer is preheated to 400 F.

2. Make a mixture of lemon juice, paprika, garlic powder, lemon pepper, and olive oil in a bowl.

3. Toss in the shrimp and coat it with the mixture.

4. Transfer the shrimp into the air fryer and cook for about 8 minutes (until the shrimp is firm and pink).

5. Serve alongside lemon slices.

68. Air Fryer Shrimp Bang

Preparation Time: 10 Minutes

Cooking Time: 30 Minutes

Servings: 4

Ingredients:

- ¼ cup sweet chili sauce
- 1 tbsp... Sriracha sauce
- ½ cup mayonnaise
- ¼ cup all-purpose flour
- 1 cup panko bread crumbs
- 1 lb raw shrimp, peeled and deveined
- 1 head loose-leaf lettuce
- 2 green onions, chopped, or to taste (optional)

Directions:

1. Make sure the setting for your Air Fryer is 400 F.

2. In a bowl, produce a blend of garlic sauce, Sriracha sauce, and mayonnaise until a flat blend. If you like, hold a certain bang source aside in a separate dipping bowl.

3. Place on a plate the flour and on another plate the panko.

4. First, dip the shrimp into the rice, and then the paste of mayonnaise. Dip it into the panko, finally.

5. On a baking sheet, transfer the coated shrimp, then into the air fryer basket without overcrowding the basket.

6. Allow them to cook for 12 minutes.

7. For the remaining shrimp, do the same.

Serve the fried shrimp with green onions in lettuce wraps as a garnish.

69. Crispy Nachos Prawns

Preparation Time: 5 Minutes

Cooking Time: 20 Minutes

Servings: 6

Ingredients:

- 18 large prawns, peeled and deveined, tails left on
- 1 egg, beaten
- 1 (10 oz.) bag nacho-cheese flavored corn chips, finely crushed

Directions:

1. Rinse the prawns and dry by patting them.

2. Get a small bowl and whisk the egg in it. Transfer the crushed chips to a separate bowl.

3. Dip a prawn in the whisked egg and the crushed chips, respectively.

4. Transfer the coated prawn to a plate and do the same for the remaining prawns.

5. Ensure that your Air Fryer is preheated to 350 F.

6. Transfer the coated prawns into the air fryer and allow to cook for 8 minutes.

7. Opaque prawns mean they are well cooked.

8. Withdraw from the air fryer and serve.

70.Coconut Pumpkin Bars

Total time: 20 min

Prep time: 10 min

Cook time: 10 min

Yield: 12 serving

Ingredients:

- 2 eggs
- 1/4 cup coconut flour
- 8 oz. pumpkin puree

- 1/2 cup coconut oil, melted
- 1/3 cup swerve
- 1 1/2 tsp. pumpkin pie spice
- 1/2 tsp. baking soda
- 1 tsp. baking powder
- Pinch of salt

Directions:

1. Place the Cuisinart oven in place 1. with the rack.
2. Beat the eggs, coconut oil, pumpkin pie spice, sweetener, and pumpkin puree in a bowl until well mixed.
3. Mix the baking powder, coconut flour, salt, and baking soda together in another dish.
4. Apply the egg mixture to the coconut flour mixture and blend properly.
5. In the prepared baking pan, add the bar mixture in and spread evenly.
6. Set to bake for 33 minutes at 350 f. Place the baking dish in the preheated oven after five minutes.
7. Slice and serve.

71.Almond Peanut Butter Bars

Total time: 40 min

Prep time: 10 min

Cook time: 30 min

Yield: 8 serving

Ingredients:

- 2 eggs
- 1/2 cup erythritol
- 1/2 cup butter softened
- 1/2 cup peanut butter

- 1 tbsp. coconut flour
- 1/2 cup almond flour

Directions:

1. Place the cuisine-style oven with the rack in place 1.
2. Toss the honey, eggs, and peanut butter together in a bowl until well mixed.
3. Add the dried ingredients and mix until the batter is smooth.
4. Spread the batter in the greased baking pan evenly.
5. Set for 35 minutes to bake at 350 f. Place the baking sheet in the preheated oven after five minutes.
6. Cut and serve.

72. Delicious Lemon Bars

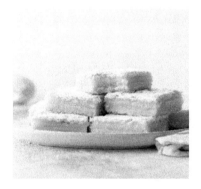

Total time: 40 min

Prep time: 10 min

Cook time: 30 min

Yield: 8 serving

Ingredients:

- 4 eggs
- 1 lemon zest
- 1/4 cup fresh lemon juice
- 1/2 cup butter softened

- 1/2 cup sour cream

- 1/3 cup erythritol

- 2 tsp. baking powder

- 2 cups almond flour

Directions:

1. Place the cuisine-style oven with the rack in place 1.

2. Whisk the eggs in a bowl until frothy.

3. Beat until well mixed, add butter and sour cream and beat.

4. Mix well with the sweetener, lemon zest, and lemon juice.

5. Add baking powder and almond flour and combine until mixed properly.

6. Move the batter and spread it evenly in a greased baking tray.

7. Set to bake for 45 minutes at 350 f. Place the baking sheet in the preheated oven after five minutes.

8. Cut and serve.

73. Easy Egg Custard

Total time: 50 min

Prep time: 10 min

Cook time: 40 min

Yield: 8 serving

Ingredients:

- 2 egg yolks

- 1 tsp. nutmeg

- 1/2 cup erythritol

- 2 cups heavy whipping cream

- 3 eggs

- 1/2 tsp. vanilla

Directions:

1. Place the Cuisinart oven in place 1. with the rack.

2. In the big mixing bowl, add all the ingredients and beat until just well mixed.

3. Pour the mixture of custard into the greased pie dish.

4. Set to bake for 40 minutes at 350 f. Place the pie dish in the preheated oven after five minutes.

5. Just serve.

74. Flavors Pumpkin Custard

Total time: 40 min

Prep time: 10 min

Cook time: 30 min

Yield: 8 serving

Ingredients:

- 4 egg yolks
- 1/2 tsp. cinnamon
- 1 tsp. liquid stevia
- 15 oz. pumpkin puree
- 3/4 cup coconut cream
- 1/8 tsp. cloves
- 1/8 tsp. ginger

Directions:

1. Place the cuisine-style oven with the rack in place 1.

2. Stir together the pumpkin puree, cloves, ginger, cinnamon, and swerve in a wide bowl.

3. Beat until well mixed, add egg yolks and beat.

4. Attach coconut cream and stir thoroughly.

5. Pour in the six ramekins with the mixture.

6. Set to bake for 45 minutes at 350 f. Place the ramekin in a preheated oven after 5 minutes.

7. Serve refrigerated and enjoy.

75. Almond Butter Cookies

Total time: 25 min

Prep time: 10 min

Cook time: 15 min

Yield: 15 serving

Ingredients:

- 1 egg
- 1/2 cup erythritol
- 1 cup almond butter
- 1 tsp. vanilla
- Pinch of salt

Directions:

1. Place the Cuisinart oven in place 1. with the rack.

2. In a big bowl, add all the ingredients and blend until well mixed.

3. Make cookies from the bowl mixture and put them on a baking pan lined with parchment.

4. Set for 20 minutes to bake at 350 f. Place the baking pan in the preheated oven after five minutes.

5. Just serve.

76.Tasty Pumpkin Cookies

Total time: 35 min

Prep time: 15 min

Cook time: 20 min

Yield: 8 serving

Ingredients:

- 1 egg
- 2 cups almond flour
- 1/2 tsp. baking powder
- 1 tsp. vanilla
- 1/2 cup butter
- 1 tsp. liquid stevia
- 1/2 tsp. pumpkin pie spice
- 1/2 cup pumpkin puree

Directions:

1. Place the Cuisinart oven in place 1. with the rack.
2. Put all the ingredients in a big bowl and blend until well mixed.
3. Make cookies from the mixture and put them on a baking sheet lined with parchment.
4. Set to bake for 30 minutes at 300 f. Place the baking dish in the preheated oven after five minutes.
5. Enjoy and serve.

77.Almond Pecan Cookies

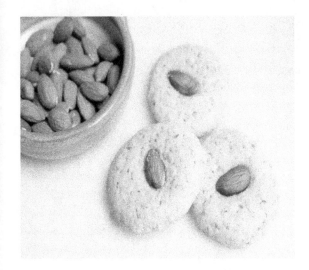

Total time: 30 min

Prep time: 10 min

Cook time: 20 min

Yield: 16 serving

Ingredients:

- 1/2 cup butter
- 1 tsp. vanilla
- 2 tsp. gelatin
- 2/3 cup swerve
- 1 cup pecans
- 1/3 cup coconut flour
- 1 cup almond flour

Directions:

1. Place the Cuisinart oven in place 1. with the rack.
2. In the food processor, add the butter, vanilla, gelatin, swerve, coconut flour, and almond flour and process until crumbs form.
3. Attach pecans and process them until they're chopped.

4. Make cookies from the prepared mixture and put them in a baking pan lined with parchment.

5. Set for 25 minutes to bake at 350 f. Place the baking pan in the preheated oven after five minutes.

6. Enjoy and serve.

78. Butter Cookies

Total time: 25 min

Prep time: 10 min

Cook time: 15 min

Yield: 24 serving

Ingredients:

- 1 egg, lightly beaten
- 1 tsp. vanilla
- 3/4 cup swerve
- 1 1/4 cups almond flour
- 1 tsp. baking powder
- 1 stick butter
- Pinch of salt

Directions:

1. Place the Cuisinart oven in place 1. with the rack.

2. Beat the butter and sweetener in a bowl until it is smooth.

3. Mix the almond flour and baking powder together in a separate dish.

4. Apply the butter mixture to the egg and vanilla and beat until smooth.

5. Apply the dry ingredients to the wet ingredients and stir until well mixed.

6. Cover the dough in plastic wrap and put it for 1 hour in the fridge.

7. Make cookies from the dough and put them on a baking sheet lined with parchment.

8. Set for 20 minutes to bake at 325 f. Place the baking pan in the preheated oven after five minutes.

9. Enjoy and serve.

79.Tasty Brownie Cookies

Total time: 30 min

Prep time: 10 min

Cook time: 20 min

Yield: 16 serving

Ingredients:

- 1 egg
- 1/2 cup erythritol
- 1/4 cup cocoa powder
- 1 cup almond butter
- 3 tbsp. milk
- 1/4 cup chocolate chips

Directions:

1. Place the Cuisinart oven in place 1. with the rack.

2. Mix the almond butter, egg, sweetener, almond milk, and cocoa powder together in a bowl until well mixed.

3. Stir in the crisps of Chocó.

4. Make cookies from the dough and put them on a baking sheet lined with parchment.

5. Set for 15 minutes to bake at 350 f. Place the baking pan in the preheated oven after five minutes.

6. Enjoy and serve.

80.Tasty Gingersnap Cookies

Total time: 20 min

Prep time: 10 min

Cook time: 10 min

Yield: 8 serving

Ingredients:

- 1 egg
- 1/2 tsp. ground cinnamon
- 1/2 tsp. ground ginger
- 1 tsp. baking powder
- 3/4 cup erythritol
- 1/2 tsp. vanilla
- 1/8 tsp. ground cloves
- 1/4 tsp. ground nutmeg
- 2/4 cup butter, melted
- 1 1/2 cups almond flour
- Pinch of salt

Directions:

1. Place the Cuisinart oven in place 1. with the rack.
2. Mix all the dried ingredients together in a mixing bowl.
3. Blend all the wet ingredients together in another tub.
4. Apply the dry ingredients to the wet ingredients and blend until the mixture is dough-like.
5. Cover and place for 30 minutes in the refrigerator.
6. Make cookies from the dough and put them on a baking sheet lined with parchment.
7. Set for 15 minutes to bake at 350 f. Place the baking pan in the preheated oven after five minutes.
8. Enjoy and serve.

81.Simple Lemon Pie

Total time: 55 min

Prep time: 25 min

Cook time: 30 min

Yield: 8 serving

Ingredients:

- 3 eggs
  - oz. butter, melted
- 3 lemon juice
- 1 lemon zest, grated
- 4 oz. erythritol
  - oz. almond flour
- Salt

Directions:

1. Place the cuisine-style oven with the rack in place 1.
2. Mix the butter, 1 oz. of sweetener, 3 oz. of almond flour, and salt together in a dish.
3. Move the dough to a pie dish and cook for 20 minutes, spreading uniformly.
4. Mix the eggs, lemon juice, lemon zest, remaining flour, sweetener and salt together in a separate dish.
5. Pour the mixture of eggs into a prepared crust.
6. Set for 35 minutes to bake at 350 f. Place the pie dish in the preheated oven after five minutes.
7. Cut and serve.

82.Flavorful Coconut Cake

Total time: 30 min

Prep time: 10 min

Cook time: 25 min

Yield: 10 servings

Ingredients:

- 5 eggs, separated
- 1/2 cup erythritol
- 1/4 cup coconut milk
- 1/2 cup coconut flour
- 1/2 tsp. baking powder
- 1/2 tsp. vanilla
- 1/2 cup butter softened
- Pinch of salt

Directions:

1. Place the cuisine-style oven with the rack in place 1.
2. Grease the buttered cake pan and set it aside.
3. Beat the sweetener and butter together in a bowl until mixed.
4. Mix well with the egg yolks, coconut milk, and vanilla.
5. Stir well and apply baking powder, coconut flour and salt.
6. Beat the egg whites in another bowl until a stiff peak emerges.
7. Fold the egg whites gently into the cake mixture.
8. In a prepared cake pan, pour batter into it.
9. Set to bake for 25 minutes at 400 f. Place the cake pans in the preheated oven for 5 minutes.
10. Cut and serve.

83.Easy Lemon Cheesecake

Total time: 55 min

Prep time: 10 min

Cook time: 35 min

Yield: 10 servings

Ingredients:

- 4 eggs
- 2 tbsp. swerve
- 1 fresh lemon juice
- 18 oz. ricotta cheese
- 1 fresh lemon zest

Directions:

1. Place the cuisine-style oven with the rack in place 1.
2. Beat the ricotta cheese in a large bowl until smooth.
3. Attach one egg at a time and whisk well.
4. Mix well with lemon juice, lemon zest, and swerve.
5. To the greased cake pan, move the mixture.
6. Set for 60 minutes to bake at 350 f. Place the cake pans in the preheated oven for 5 minutes.
7. Cut and serve.

84.Lemon Butter Cake

Total time: 55 min

Prep time: 20 min

Cook time: 35 min

Yield: 10 servings

Ingredients:

- 4 eggs
- 1/2 cup butter softened
- 2 tsp. baking powder
- 1/4 cup coconut flour
- 2 cups almond flour
- 2 tbsp. lemon zest
- 1/2 cup fresh lemon juice
- 1/4 cup erythritol

- 1 tbsp. vanilla

Directions:

1. Place the Cuisinart oven in place 1. with the rack.
2. Whisk all the ingredients in a wide bowl until a smooth batter is created.
3. Fill the loaf pan with butter.
4. Set to bake for 60 minutes at 300 f. Place the loaf pan in the preheated oven after five minutes.
5. Slicing and serving.

85.Cream Cheese Butter Cake

Total time: 45 min

Prep time: 10 min

Cook time: 35 min

Yield: 10 servings

Ingredients:

- 5 eggs
- 1 cup swerve
- 4 oz. cream cheese, softened
- 1 tsp. vanilla
- 1 tsp. orange extract
- 1 tsp. baking powder
- oz. almond flour
- 1/2 cup butter, softened

Directions:

1. Place the cuisine-style oven with the rack in place 1.
2. In the mixing bowl, add all the ingredients and whisk until fluffy.
3. Pour the batter into a cake pan that has been prepared.

4. Set for 40 minutes to bake at 350 f. Place the cake pans in the preheated oven for 5 minutes.

5. Slice and serve

86.Easy Ricotta Cake

Total time: 55 min

Prep time: 20 min

Cook time: 35 min

Yield: 8 servings

Ingredients:

- 2 eggs
- 1/2 cup erythritol
- 1/4 cup coconut flour
- 15 oz. ricotta
- Pinch of salt

Directions:

1. Place the cuisine-style oven with the rack in place 1.
2. Mix the eggs in a dish.
3. Connect the remaining ingredients and blend until well mixed.
4. Apply the batter to the greased cake tray.
5. Set to bake for 50 minutes at 350 f. Place the cake pans in the preheated oven for 5 minutes.
6. Cut and serve.

87.Strawberry Muffins

Total time: 45 min

Prep time: 10 min

Cook time: 35 min

Yield: 10 servings

Ingredients:

- 4 eggs
- 1/4 cup water
- 1/2 cup butter, melted
- 2 tsp. baking powder
- 2 cups almond flour
- 2/3 cup strawberries, chopped
- 2 tsp. vanilla
- 1/4 cup erythritol
- Pinch of salt

Directions:

1. Place the Cuisinart oven in place 1. with the rack.
2. Line and set aside 12-cups of a muffin tin with cupcake liners.
3. Mix the almond flour, baking powder, and salt together in a medium dish.
4. Whisk the eggs, sweetener, vanilla, water, and butter together in a separate cup.
5. Apply the mixture of almond flour to the egg mixture and stir until well mixed.
6. Attach the strawberries and stir thoroughly.
7. Pour the batter into the muffin tin that has been packed.
8. Set for 25 minutes to bake at 350 f. Place the muffin tin in the preheated oven for 5 minutes.
9. Enjoy and serve.

88. Mini Brownie Muffins

Total time: 35 min

Prep time: 10 min

Cook time: 25 min

Yield: 10 servings

Ingredients:

- 3 eggs
- 1/2 cup swerve
- 1 cup almond flour
- 1 tbsp. gelatin
- 1/3 cup butter, melted
- 1/3 cup cocoa powder

Directions:

1. Place the Cuisinart oven in place 1. with the rack.
2. Set aside and line 6-cups of a muffin tin with cupcake liners.
3. In the mixing bowl, add all ingredients and stir until well mixed.
4. In the prepared muffin pan, pour the mixture into it.
5. Set for 20 minutes to bake at 350 f. Place the muffin tin in the preheated oven for 5 minutes.
6. Enjoy and serve.

89.Cinnamon Cheesecake Bars

Total time: 35 min

Prep time: 10 min

Cook time: 25 min

Yield: 10 servings

Ingredients:

- Nonstick cooking spray
- 16 oz. Cream cheese, soft
- 1 tsp. vanilla
- 1 ¼ cups sugar, divided
- 2 tubes refrigerated crescent rolls
- 1 tsp. cinnamon
- ¼ cup butter

Directions:

1. Place the rack in position 1. Using cooking spray to spray the bottom of an 8x11-inch pan.

2. Beat the cream cheese, vanilla, and 3⁄4 cup sugar in a medium bowl until smooth.

3. On the bottom of the prepared pan, roll out one can of crescent rolls, close the perforations, and press the sides partway up.

4. Spread the mixture of cream cheese uniformly over the crescents.

5. Roll out the second can of crescents, covering the perforations over the top of the cheese mixture.

6. Stir the cinnamon and the remaining sugar together in a small cup. Let the butter melt.

7. Set the oven to 375 °F for 35 minutes to bake.

8. Sprinkle over the top of the crescents with the cinnamon sugar and drizzle with melted butter.

9. Place the pan in the oven after the oven has preheated for 5 minutes, then bake for 30 minutes until the top is golden brown.

10. Absolutely cool. Before slicing and serving, cover and refrigerate for at least 2 hours.

90.Strawberry Cobbler

Total time: 35 min

Prep time: 10 min

Cook time: 25 min

Yield: 10 servings

Ingredients:

- Butter flavored cooking spray
- 2 tbsp. Cornstarch
- ¼ cup fresh lemon juice

- ½ cup + 1 tbsp. Sugar divided
- 3 cups strawberries, hulled & sliced
- 5 tbsp. Butter, cold & diced
- 1 cup flour
- 1 ½ tsp. baking powder
- ½ tsp. salt
- ½ cup heavy cream

Directions:

1. Place the rack in position 1. Using cooking spray to spray a 9-inch baking pan.

2. Combine the cornstarch, lemon juice, and half a cup of sugar in a saucepan. Cook, constantly stirring, over medium heat, until the sugar dissolves and the mixture thickens.

3. Remove from the heat and stir in the berries gently. Pour 2 teaspoons of butter into a prepared pan and sprinkle.

4. Combine the flour, remaining sugar, baking powder, and salt in a large bowl. Split the remaining butter using a fork or pastry cutter until the mixture resembles coarse crumbs.

5. Stir in the cream and sprinkle the strawberries over them.

6. Set the oven to 400 degrees F for 30 minutes to bake. Place the cobbler in the oven after five minutes and bake for 25 minutes until bubbly and golden brown. Let cool 10 minutes prior to serving, at least.

91.Baked Zucchini Fries

Total time: 20 min

Prep time: 10 min

Cook time: 10 min

Yield: 4 servings

Ingredients:

- 3 medium zucchinis, sliced lengthwise

- 1/2 cup of
- 2 egg, the white part
- 1/4 teaspoon of garlic powder
- 2 tablespoons of parmesan cheese, grated
- Salt and pepper to taste

Directions

1. Whisk the egg whites together in a bowl and season with salt and pepper.
2. In a separate dish, combine the garlic powder, breadcrumbs, and cheese together.
3. Dip the zucchini sticks into one after the other of the egg, bread crumb and cheese mixture, then place the Air Fryer tray on a single layer.
4. Coat lightly with cooking spray and bake for about 15 minutes at 390 °F until golden brown.
5. Serve with a marinara sauce for dipping.

92.Roasted Heirloom Tomato with Baked Feta

Total time: 20 min

Prep time: 10 min

Cook time: 10 min

Yield: 4 servings

Ingredients:

For the Tomato:

- 2 heirloom tomatoes, sliced thickly into½ inch circular slices
- 1 8-ounceof feta cheese, sliced thickly into½ inch circular slices
- ½ cup of red onions, sliced thinly
- 1 pinch of salt
- 1 tablespoon of olive oil

For the Basil Pesto:

- ½ cup of basil, chopped roughly
- ½cup of parsley, roughly chopped
- 3 tablespoons of pine nuts, toasted
- ½ cup of parmesan cheese, grated
- 1 garlic clove
- 1 pinch of salt
- ½ cup of olive oil

Directions:

1. Start by making pesto. To do this, a food processor mixes garlic, parmesan, parsley, toasted pine nuts, basil, and salt.

2. Turn it on and eventually apply the olive oil to the pesto. Store and place in the refrigerator until finished, before ready to use.

3. Preheat the 390 ° F Air Fryer. Pat a dried tomato with a towel on paper. Spread a tablespoon of the pesto on top of each tomato slice and top with the feta. Add the red onions and toss with 1 tablespoon of olive oil; put on top of the feta.

4. In the cooking bowl, put the feta/ tomatoes and cook until the feta is brownish and begins to soften, or 12 to 14 minutes.

5. Add 1 spoonful of basil pesto and a tablespoon of salt. Enjoy and serve.

93.Garam Masala Beans

Total time: 20 min

Prep time: 10 min

Cook time: 10 min

Yield: 4 servings

Ingredients:

- 9-ounce of Beans
- 2 Eggs
- 1/2 cup of breadcrumbs

- 1/2 cup of flour
- 1/2 teaspoon of garam masala
- 2 teaspoon of chili powder
- Olive Oil
- Salt to taste

Directions:

1. At 350°F, preheat the Air Fryer. In a cup, combine the chili powder, garam masala, flour, and salt, and stir well. Place the eggs in one hand and beat them.

2. On a different pan, pour the breadcrumbs and then cover the beans with the flour mixture. Now dip the beans in the mixture of the eggs and then the breadcrumbs. For all the beans, do this.

3. Place the beans and cook for 4 minutes in the Air Fryer tray. Open and coat the oil on the beans and simmer again for another 3 minutes. Serve it hot.

94.Crisp Potato Wedges

Total time: 20 min

Prep time: 10 min

Cook time: 10 min

Yield: 4 servings

Ingredients:

- 3 teaspoons of olive oil
- 2 big potatoes
- ¼ cup of sweet chili sauce
- ¼ cup of sour cream

Directions:

1. To build a wedge shape, slice the potatoes lengthwise.

2. Hot the 356 ° F Air Fryer.

3. In a bowl, put the wedges and add the oil. Toss gently until the oil is thoroughly coated with the potatoes.

4. Place the side of the skin facing down into the cooking basket and cook for about 15 minutes. Toss, then cook until golden brown for another 10 minutes.

5. Best eaten with chili and sour cream when warm.

95. Crispy Onion Rings

Total time: 20 min

Prep time: 10 min

Cook time: 10 min

Yield: 4 servings

Ingredients:

- 1 big of sized onion, thinly sliced
- 8 ounces of milk
- 1 egg
- 6 ounces of breadcrumbs
- 1 teaspoon of baking powder
- 10 ounces of flour
- 1 teaspoon of salt

Directions:

1. Heat your Air Fryer to 360°F for 10 minutes.

2. Detach the onion slices to separate rings.

3. Mix the baking powder, flour, and salt in a bowl.

4. Put the onion rings into the flour mixture to coat them. Beat the egg and the milk and stir into the flour to form a batter. Dip the flour-coated rings in the batter.

5. Put the breadcrumbs in a small tray, place the onion rings in it, and ensure all sides are well coated.

6. Place the rings in the fryer basket and air fry for 10 minutes until crisp.

96.Cheese Lasagna and Pumpkin Sauce

Total time: 20 min

Prep time: 10 min

Cook time: 10 min

Yield: 2 servings

Ingredients:

- 25 ounces of pumpkin, peeled and finely chopped
- 4 teaspoons of finely chopped rosemary
- 17½ ounces of beets, cooked and thinly sliced
- 1medium-sized onion, chopped
- 1 cup of goat's cheese, grated
- Grana Padano cheese, grated
- 28 ounces of tomatoes, cubed
- 6 teaspoons of olive oil
- 8½ounces of lasagna sheets

Directions:

1. In a cup, mix the pumpkin, 3 teaspoons of oil, and rosemary and fry for 10 minutes at 347 degrees F.

2. To mix the rosemary, peppers, and onions into a puree, remove the pumpkin from the Air Fryer and use a hand blender. In a saucepan, pour the puree and put it over low heat for 5 minutes.

3. Grease a dish that is heatproof with grease. First, put the pumpkin sauce and then the lasagna sheets in. Divide the sauce into two, and the goat cheese and beets into three. Put on the lasagna a portion of the beets and sauce and top with a portion of the goat cheese. Repeat this until all the ingredients are used, and you finish it with cheese and sauce.

4. Add the lasagna and air fried the Grana Padano at 300 ° F for 45 minutes. Detach and allow to cool.

5. Using a cookie cutter to cut out circular shapes and roast for 6 minutes at 390 ° F. Garnish with the goats' grated cheese and beet slices.

97.Pasta Wraps

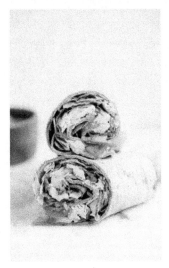

Total time: 20 min

Prep time: 10 min

Cook time: 10 min

Yield: 2 servings

Ingredients:

- 8 ounces of flour
- 2 ounces of pasta
- 6 teaspoons of olive oil
- 1 clove of garlic, chopped
- 1 green chili, chopped
- 1 small onion, chopped
- 1 tablespoon of tomato pastes
- ½ teaspoon of garam masala
- Salt to taste

Directions:

1. Mix the flour with water and salt to make a dough. Add 1teaspoon of the oil mixture and set aside.

2. Put the pasta in boiling water and add 3 teaspoons of oil and salt to it. Drain excess water when cooked.

3. Sauté the onions, garlic, chili, and add the spices, salt, and tomato paste. Lastly, add the cooked pasta and cover with a lid and turn down the heat to low.

4. Preheat the Air fryer to 390°F.

5. Mold the dough into small balls; flatten them using a rolling pin into a circle. Put the pasta stuffing on them and fold the opposite edges together—seal edges with water.

6. Place into the Air Fryer and cook for 15 minutes until golden. Remove and serve while hot with a sauce.

98.Homemade Tater Tots

Total time: 20 min

Prep time: 10 min

Cook time: 10 min

Yield: 2 servings

Ingredients:

- 1 medium-sized russet potato, chopped
- 1 teaspoon of ground onion
- 1 teaspoon of vegetable oil
- ½ teaspoon of ground black pepper
- Salt to taste

Directions:

1. Boil the potatoes until they are a little more like al dente. Drain the water, add the onions, oil, and pepper and mash with the mixture.

2. Preheat the 379 ° F Air Fryer.

3. Mold the potatoes into tater tots with the mash. Place the fryer in the air and bake for eight minutes. Shake the tots and bake for a further 5 minutes.

99.Mushroom, Onion, and Feta Frittata

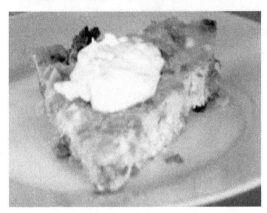

Total time: 20 min

Prep time: 10 min

Cook time: 10 min

Yield: 2 serving

Ingredients:

- 4 cups of button mushrooms, cleaned and cut thinly into¼ inch
- 6eggs
- 1 red onion, peeled and sliced thinly into¼ an inch
- 6 tablespoons of feta cheese, crumbled
- 2 tablespoons of olive oil
- 1 pinch of salt

Directions

1. In a sauté pan, apply the olive oil and swirl the onions and mushrooms about until tender under medium pressure. Remove from the heat on a dry kitchen towel and cool.
2. Preheat the 330°F Air Fryer. A touch of salt is added to whisk the eggs thoroughly in a mixing Bowland.

3. The inside and bottom of an 8-in suit. Slightly heat tolerant baking dish with mist. Through the baking bowl, pour the whisked eggs, apply the onion and mushroom mixture and then add the cheese.

4. Place the dish in the cooking basket and cook in the Air Fryer for 27 to 30 minutes or until a knife inserted in the middle of the frittata comes out clean.

100. Roasted Bell Pepper Vegetable Salad

Total time: 20 min

Prep time: 10 min

Cook time: 10 min

Yield: 2 serving

Ingredients:

- 1½ ounces of yogurt
- 1 medium-sized red bell pepper
- 2ounces of rocket leaves
- 3 teaspoons of lime juice
- 1 romaine lettuce
- 1 ounce of olive oil
- Ground black pepper and salt to taste

Directions:

1. Heat the Air-Fryer to 392 degrees F and put the bell pepper in it. Roast until a little charred for 10 minutes. Put the pepper in a dish, cover it, and leave for 15 minutes or so.

2. Divide the bell pepper into four parts, remove the skin and seeds and cut the pepper into thin strips.

3. In a bowl, carefully mix the lime juice, olive oil, and yogurt together. As needed, add the salt and pepper and stir.

4. Add the yogurt mixture to the rocket beans, broccoli, and pepper strips and toss to combine.

Conclusion

Air fryers are amazing both for food and health. This book is a compilation of amazing breakfast, lunch, meat, vegetarian, snack and dessert recipes that you can prepare at home using an air fryer and relish with your family.

9 781802 162967